W9-BSS-241

Old-Fashioned Cures and Proven Home Remedies

That Lower Your Cholesterol and Blood Pressure, Improve Your Memory, and Keep Diabetes and Arthritis Under Control

Publisher's Note

The editors of FC&A have taken careful measures to ensure the accuracy and usefulness of the information in this book. While every attempt was made to assure accuracy, some Web sites, addresses, telephone numbers, and other information may have changed since printing.

This book is intended for general information only. It does not constitute medical advice or practice. We cannot guarantee the safety or effectiveness of any treatment or advice mentioned. Readers are urged to consult with their health care professionals and get their approval before undertaking therapies suggested by information in this book, keeping in mind that errors in the text may occur as in all publications and that new findings may supercede older information.

"Bear one another's burdens, and thereby fulfill the law of Christ. So then, while we have opportunity, let us do good to all people, and especially to those who are of the household of the faith."

Galatians 6:2,10

FC&A Medical Publishing®
103 Clover Green
Peachtree City, GA 30269

Produced by the staff of FC&A

ISBN 978-1-932470-75-8

Contents

Contents

Contents

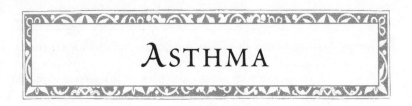

Asthma

Practical advice to help you breathe better

Would you be willing to kiss a frog to cure your asthma? That's all you have to do, according to an old Texas folk remedy. Breathe into a frog's mouth before daylight, and the frog will die before sundown and take your asthma with it. You will never be bothered again.

Wouldn't it be nice if it could be that easy? (Or, maybe not so easy, depending on your view of frogs!) Unfortunately, asthma is one of those chronic conditions that hangs on despite your best efforts. It's caused by a faulty immune system, although allergies, family history, and poor air quality may also be involved. You can have a mild case that you seldom notice, or it can be a constant and frightening companion.

When something triggers an asthma attack, the smooth muscles around your bronchial tubes tighten up and stay tight, shrinking your airways. Then inflammation swells those airways and fills them with mucus. You cough, wheeze, and are short of breath. It takes specific medicines to fight severe asthma, and even with moderate or intermittent asthma, you need your doctor's advice.

But the way you eat and live can make a big difference in the way asthma affects your life. Foods and supplements can protect you from inflammation, bolster your immune system, and help open up your airways. Eliminating asthma triggers inside your home and staying away from the ones outside can cut down on the number of attacks as well.

Warm, moist air from a vaporizer helps limit winter asthma attacks, but don't let humidity in your house get above 40 percent.

In the summer, keep humidity below 50 percent with a dehumidifier or air conditioner, which also filters out pollen and other allergens.

At least half the people with asthma also have gastroesophageal reflux disease (GERD). It's not clear if one causes the other, but you may clear up asthma symptoms just by taking antacids for your heartburn.

Read on to discover more practical, homespun advice for easing asthma's effects. And it won't involve kissing frogs – promise.

Carotenoids: superstar asthma fighters

The best game plan for fighting asthma is a healthy diet, and the key players in that plan are antioxidants – especially carotenoids. These powerful food stars keep your lungs working their best by bolstering your immunity and fending off inflammation.

Carotenoids give foods a rich yellow, orange, or red color and are found in deeply pigmented fruits and vegetables like apricots, carrots, cantaloupe, sweet potatoes, and tomatoes. Leafy green vegetables like spinach and lettuce are a prime source of other antioxidants.

A study that questioned 68,535 French women found those who ate the most tomatoes, carrots, and leafy vegetables were less likely

MythBuster: Hold the caffeine?

Caffeine may be bad for a lot of things, but not for asthma. In fact, drinking one or two cups of coffee or tea at the start of an attack could stop it from escalating. Caffeine is chemically related to the drug theophylline, a key ingredient in asthma medications. It helps relax your bronchial tubes and, according to one study, may improve your breathing for up to four hours.

to have asthma. An Australian study found fewer carotenoids in the blood of people with asthma than in those who didn't have it.

For asthma sufferers, beta carotene takes top billing among the more than 600 carotenoids. Your body converts beta carotene to vitamin A, which helps regulate your immune system and maintain the lining of your respiratory tract.

Apples keep asthma at bay

The old saying about apples keeping the doctor away is true. An apple is a wonderful snack made to order for avoiding asthma. You don't even need one every day. Just a couple of apples a week lowers your asthma risk, and five a week makes a big improvement in the amount of air your lungs can take in. Apples won't eliminate your asthma, but they'll sure help you breathe easier while you're trying to avoid it.

Experts believe quercetin and other flavonoids are the phytochemicals that boost your lung power the most. Apples seem to have a secret formula, however. Onions, tea, and red wine are also rich in flavonoids, but they don't improve your breathing ability as well as apples. More nutrients are in the apple peel than the flesh, so be sure and eat the whole thing.

5 top nutrients for healthy lungs

A few favorite foods aren't enough to keep asthma from getting you down. You need a broad and balanced diet for good lung health. Here are some important vitamins and minerals you should include in your diet. It's always best to get nutrients from the food you eat, but sometimes it doesn't hurt to take extra supplements. Just be sure and discuss it with your doctor. Some supplements, like vitamin D and magnesium, can be deadly if you take too much.

Vitamin C. The major antioxidant in your airways is vitamin C. It's no wonder people with low vitamin C intake are more likely to have asthma. Five servings of fruits and vegetables a day give you the precious C you need – about 220 milligrams (mg). Short-term studies show you can get extra benefits with daily supplemental doses of 500 mg to 1,000 mg.

Vitamin E. Another powerful antioxidant, vitamin E has been shown to help seniors' lungs in particular. It is often used along with vitamin C, and experts sometimes are not sure which one provides the most benefit. You can get vitamin E from vegetable oils, fruits, vegetables, wheat germ, soybeans, and grain products.

Vitamin D. Steroids are an important treatment for asthma, but they don't work for some people. British scientists think low levels of vitamin D may be the reason. A test-tube study found that adding vitamin D3 to cultures of T-cells improved responsiveness to steroids. Other experts believe vitamin D also helps overall lung function, especially for people over age 60. Your body makes most of your vitamin D from sunlight since it's not found in many foods. If you don't get out much, you can take up to 400 IU – 600 if you're over age 70 – in daily supplements.

Magnesium. Emergency room doctors may use magnesium to stop severe asthma attacks. It's a natural bronchodilator that helps open up your airways. Most people don't get enough magnesium in their diets, but those who do have fewer problems with asthma. It's found in spinach, avocados, legumes, and oysters.

Selenium. Another key mineral in asthma control, selenium stops inflammation and helps protect the cells of your lungs. People with more selenium in their diets seem to have less asthma. Find it in enriched grain, walnuts, tuna, and beef, or take 55 micrograms a day as a supplement.

Lose weight to lose breathing problems

Shed your excess pounds and you'll breathe better. You may still have asthma, but then again, you may find out you never had it in

Music gives two-toned relief

A little Beethoven or Tony Bennett may be just the ticket to relieving your asthma. When stress and anxiety trigger symptoms, turn to your favorite music for help with relaxing. It's a proven stress reducer. Music also may prove to be a weapon for fighting asthma. Researchers are studying how blowing into wind instruments like flutes and horns can build up your lungs.

the first place. Sounds confusing, but some experts believe obesity creates the same symptoms as asthma. They suspect that many overweight people think they have asthma when they are just suffering from obesity-related breathing problems.

Here's how it works. Obesity makes it difficult to breathe. Your lungs are crowded into a smaller space and your respiratory muscles have to work harder. You wheeze, are short of breath, and have less lung capacity – the same as if you had asthma.

Obese people have low-grade inflammation that tightens up the smooth muscles around the airways and makes them smaller, just like asthma does. A hormone that causes asthma-related inflammation increases in fat tissue and one that is anti-inflammatory decreases.

Losing weight improves all those conditions. If you have asthma, you shouldn't have it as bad. And if you couldn't breathe simply because you were overweight, you may be rid of the problem altogether.

Tasty seasonings open your airways

Fruits and vegetables aren't the only things you can eat to ease asthma. Herbal garnishes and seasonings can provide relief, too.

Pop in some parsley. The world's most popular herb delivers potent antioxidant power from large amounts of vitamin C and beta carotene. Use it in soups, stews, salads, and sandwiches. And don't forget to eat the decorative parsley on your dinner plate. It not only helps your breathing, it freshens your breath, too.

Remember rosemary. You'll also find plenty of antioxidants in this pungent herb. In folk medicine, rosemary is an antispasmodic and respiratory cure. Prepare it as a tea for asthma relief. Rosemary is a wonderful seasoning for vegetables and legumes and is especially tasty on chicken or pork.

Rosemary

3 herbal helpers to try

People all over the world use herbal remedies to treat asthma and many other conditions. You won't find doctors prescribing them in the United States, though. Herbs are classified as dietary supplements so they are not regulated by the Food and Drug Administration. That means you have no assurance of their quality or effectiveness. If you want to try them, make sure you get standardized extracts. Here are a few herbal remedies to think about.

Ginkgo biloba. Mostly known for helping people with dementia and Alzheimer's disease, ginkgo is also helpful for asthma, studies show. It's relatively safe, but it may increase bleeding time so you shouldn't take it with warfarin, aspirin, or other anticoagulants.

Boswellia serrata. This tree-bark extract has anti-inflammatory powers. It can reduce the number of attacks for people with mild asthma who take it for four to eight weeks. Boswellia is considered safe with few side effects when taken as directed.

Butterbur. Studies from Europe claim certain butterbur extracts are safe and effective for both asthma and hay fever. The most widely tested and used butterbur extract is Petadolex. Avoid supplements containing whole butterbur since some parts of the plant are poisonous or may cause cancer.

Avoid double whammy from allergy triggers

Aa-choo! Once you start sneezing, prepare yourself because an asthma attack may be close behind.

Any kind of allergen – including dust mites, air pollution, and pets – can set off an attack that leaves you gasping for air. Head off this double whammy of allergy and asthma triggers by knowing where allergens hide.

- Automobile drivers' seats, chairs and sofas, and carpets can all be huge reservoirs of dust mite residue and dog and cat allergens, even if you don't own a pet.
- Bed pillows can harbor fungus spores that trigger asthma attacks. Researchers found 16 different fungi in pillows used between 18 months and 20 years. Synthetic materials are the worst, so use feather pillows, and have them disinfected regularly.
- Gas cooking stoves produce nitrogen dioxide, which is another trigger. If you have asthma and cook with gas, consider an electric range.

Control asthma with sensible exercise

Exercise isn't a bad thing if you have asthma. Once you get your doctor's OK, you can actually help control asthma with long-term exercise. The American Thoracic Society recommends moderate aerobic exercise for asthma.

But you do need to make wise choices in setting up your fitness program. Exercise also can trigger an asthma attack, especially if you have exercise-induced asthma (EIA). Here are some tips to help.

- If you run, use an indoor track to avoid outdoor pollutants.

- Swimming is an excellent exercise because it gives you moist air to breathe and a good aerobic workout.
- Yoga has particular benefits for people with asthma. Its slow, controlled movements and deep breathing exercises not only open up your lungs but may also reduce inflammation that occurs with asthma.
- Don't work out in the evening, when your lungs may have more problems functioning.
- Always include warm-up and cool-down periods in your routine.

EIA is a limited form of asthma that affects mostly children and young adults. You are more likely to experience it with regular-paced activity – like running – in cold, dry air. Try breathing through a scarf or your nose to warm up your airways. To prevent flare-ups, look for activities that require short bursts of exercise, like tennis or softball, instead of long-duration stamina like distance running and cycling.

Slow breathing opens airways

Remember how you learned to pucker up and kiss? Well, now you can use the same move to help control your asthma. Pursed lip breathing helps you learn to empty your lungs, which keeps your airways from narrowing. It also helps strengthen the muscles you use to breathe.

Follow these steps several times a day. They may take some practice, but eventually they should feel as natural as kissing your favorite grandchild. You can then use the technique whenever you feel stressed or have problems breathing.

- Inhale through your nose to warm and moisten the air. Each breath should take about two seconds.
- Purse your lips like you are kissing, then exhale slowly. Don't force the air out. Just blow gently for about four to six seconds.

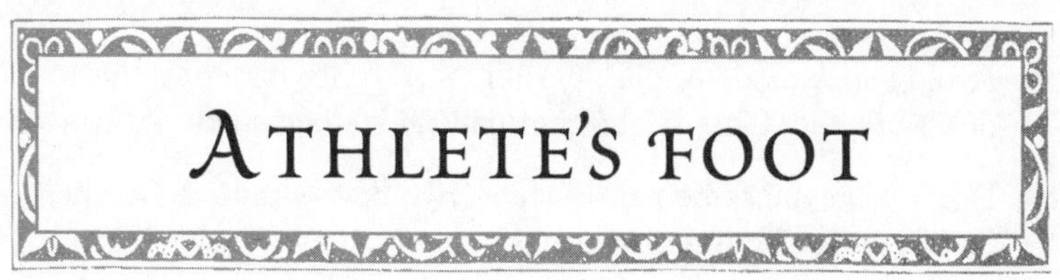

Athlete's Foot

Simple steps make happy feet

There's a whole kingdom of organisms in the plant world called fungi. Most are harmless, even helpful – like yeasts or mushrooms. Others, like mold, can turn a good slice of bread bad, or, in the case of *Penicillium*, save a life.

Some fungi can live and work in your body and, if you're healthy, are controlled by your own immune system and other fungi. If, however, your immune system isn't operating at peak power, you could be susceptible to certain fungi that can't wait to move in and make trouble.

That's the story behind tinea pedis, commonly known as athlete's foot or ringworm of the feet. You don't have to be an athlete to suffer from this annoying condition. In fact, experts aren't sure exactly why some people become infected and others don't. But if you are susceptible, and you come in contact with a particular fungus, you can develop dry, scaly patches of skin on your feet and toes; itching; blisters; or burning. Your first step is to get a diagnosis from your doctor, and if you suffer from diabetes, don't try to self-treat.

Athlete's foot can last a long time and may come and go, so people have tried all kinds of remedies – some a little crazier than others. Experts will tell you not to bother tying a string around your toes or wrapping your feet in brown paper. They'll tell you the most important thing to do to prevent and treat athlete's foot is keep your feet clean and dry because the fungus doesn't survive well in this type of environment.

- Wash your feet every day, and be sure to dry them well – including between your toes.

- Avoid shoes made of plastic, rubber, or other materials that don't breathe. Choose shoes of natural leather, suede, or canvas.
- Don't wear the same pair of shoes two days in a row. Let them dry for a day between wearings.
- Avoid socks made of synthetic materials that don't breathe. Pick socks of cotton or wool instead.
- Remember the "socks first" rule. To avoid spreading athlete's foot fungus from your feet to your groin area, put on your socks before your underwear.

The same fungus that causes athlete's foot can also cause toenail fungus, but the treatments are different. The *Nail problems* chapter offers some home remedies for toenail fungus.

Double trouble for foot fungus

Athlete's foot fungus is something like the mythical vampire of folklore: it hates sunlight and garlic. Sounds strange, but you can fight this pesky condition with these two home remedies. Researchers had soldiers with athlete's foot compare a gel made from garlic extract to terbinafine (Lamisil), a common drug used to kill the fungus. Both treatments worked equally well, confirming garlic's antifungal properties.

To try this remedy at home, make a paste of mashed garlic and oil and rub on athlete's foot spots. You can also dust your feet with garlic powder or cut up raw garlic and put in your shoes. How does sunlight affect athlete's foot? Since fungus thrives in damp places, it hates to see the light of day. Fight the itchies by putting your shoes on the windowsill when you're not wearing them or going barefoot in the sunlight.

Tea tree-tment powers away the itch

Reach for tea tree oil when the discomfort of athlete's foot proves just too much. This ancient Australian remedy is a natural

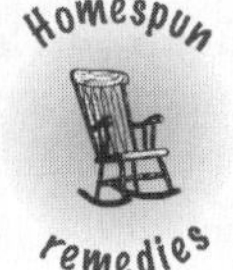

Soothing soaks battle itchy-feet blues

Itching and irritation can make even a mild case of athlete's foot hard to live with. Fight the itch by soaking your feet in a soothing bath. See if one of these homespun remedies does the trick for you.

- **Vinegar.** Make a foot soak of equal parts vinegar and warm water. Or simply add two cups of vinegar to your regular bath water.
- **Salt.** Mix 4 teaspoons of table salt into a quart of warm water.
- **Black tea.** Steep five tea bags in a quart of warm water.

Soak your feet for about 10 minutes and finish by drying them completely – especially between your toes. Try a blow dryer on the lowest heat setting to get this done quickly.

antifungal agent that clears up symptoms just as well as tolnaftate, the generic name for Tinactin, a common over-the-counter cream. You'll have to go with the commercial medicine if you want to actually kill the fungus, but for quick relief, use a few drops of tea tree oil in an aromatic footbath, dilute it in vinegar and dab on your toes with a cloth, or add it to a natural foot powder.

Handy no-sweat foot remedies

The average foot has 250,000 sweat glands, producing about 8 ounces of sweat every day. This constant moisture creates a breeding ground for the fungus that causes athlete's foot. To help keep those pups dry, rub on some diaper rash cream containing zinc oxide. Or spray antiperspirant on the soles of your feet.

Fragrant soak soothes athlete's foot misery

The itching, burning, and scaliness of athlete's foot fungus can be annoying and long-lasting. To take the edge off your symptoms, try soaking your feet in an aromatic foot bath containing tea tree oil, which kills fungus, and peppermint and sage essential oils which may help with itching.

- 3 drops peppermint oil
- 5 drops sage oil
- 5 drops tea tree oil

Fill a basin with water that is comfortably warm. Mix in the oils, and soak your feet for about 15 minutes. Dry them completely, since damp skin allows the fungus to grow. Remember – don't put full-strength essential oils directly on your skin.

MythBuster: Is barefoot best?

Many believe you can "catch" athlete's foot by going barefoot. It's true certain susceptible people can pick up the fungus if they go barefoot in public locker rooms or near pools with wet floors. So wear sandals or shoes in those areas. But going barefoot in other places doesn't lead to athlete's foot. In fact, experts say going shoeless at home is a good idea. Let your feet air out – and keep them free and clear of fungus – by adopting the ancient custom of going barefoot in the house. You can keep your floors clean, give your vacuum a break, and cool your feet at the same time.

BACK PAIN

Smart strategies save your spine

Your back does a lot of – well, backbreaking work. It keeps you upright, carries your weight, protects the bundle of nerves known as your spinal cord, plus gives you the strength to lift heavy items and the flexibility to bend, twist, and turn.

To do all this, it uses 33 – count 'em, 33 – separate bones, joined together like puzzle pieces that hinge and move. Between each bone, or vertebra, is a spongy cushion filled with water. With age and stress, the edges of these fluid-filled discs get thinner, making them more likely to bulge out, or herniate, and press on the nerves in your spinal cord. The discs also dry out, so your bony vertebrae start rubbing together. Plus, your back muscles weaken with age, making it easier to "overdo" once-simple tasks like lifting groceries or bending in the garden.

Put it all together, and it's no wonder 80 percent of people are laid low with back problems at some point in their lives. Most cases aren't serious. Nine out of 10 get better in about six weeks with little or no treatment. However, you should see a doctor immediately if you:

- hurt so badly you can't move.
- have pain shooting down your leg to below your knee.
- feel any numbness, tingling, or weakness, particularly in your legs.
- hurt worse when lying down or at night.
- lose control over bladder or bowel functions.
- suddenly and unintentionally start to lose weight.

- still don't feel better after two or three weeks.

Otherwise, at-home self-care may be all you need to get on your feet. Take over-the-counter pain relievers like ibuprofen or acetaminophen short-term to ease pain and soothe inflammation. And avoid bending and lifting heavy items for the first six weeks after hurting yourself. Of course, the best advice is to avoid getting hurt in the first place. These three tips can help guard your back.

Get in shape. Being overweight and out of shape definitely boosts your risk of back problems. Tone up and drop those extra pounds with some moderate exercise. Water aerobics are especially good if you are overweight or have bad joints.

Kick the nicotine habit. Smoking is a major risk factor for back pain because nicotine restricts the blood supply that feeds your spinal discs, making them slower to heal.

Lift and carry carefully. Picking up heavy items the wrong way puts stress on your spine and doubles your risk of a herniated disc. Keep your back straight and squat. Use your leg muscles – not your back – to lift, and carry objects close to your body. Don't turn while lifting.

MythBuster: Is bed rest best?

A growing number of doctors believe staying active is better for a back injury than bed rest. Out of more than 1,000 people with back pain, those who kept bed rest and pain medicine to a minimum recovered faster than those prescribed drugs and confined to bed. Extended bed rest actually weakens your muscles, which can slow recovery. Rest for the first day or two if necessary, but get up and move around a few minutes each hour. Most of all, get back to your normal activities as soon as you're able.

Next up, learn natural ways to help your body repair itself, including specific foods, nutrients, exercises, and savvy tips.

Fire and ice bounce you back fast

You have to move quickly to heal a hurt back. Take these steps as soon as you injure yourself, and you'll be back on your feet in no time.

- Ice down the injury for up to 20 minutes every two hours for the first two or three days. The cold numbs pain and cuts blood flow, staunching swelling and internal bleeding. For fast, cheap relief, try an ice pack, a bag of frozen vegetables, or even an ice cube massage.
- Switch to heat therapy after the first two or three days. Heat opens up your blood vessels allowing more oxygen to the injured area and calming muscle spasms. Use a heating pad for 20 to 30 minutes, enjoy a hot shower, or soak in a warm bath.

Exercise gets your back back on track

You may not want to get off the couch if your back hurts, but you probably should. Exercise can work wonders for chronic back pain, but experts don't always agree what kind is best.

Some studies show a combination of stretching and strengthening exercises work well for chronic low back pain. Stretching muscles eases pain, while building strength can help you function better.

Other experts say forget about specific back exercises. Just get up and move. People with chronic low back pain in a new study actually fared better doing general activities like walking and swimming. Those who did specific back exercises, on the other hand, reported more pain and disability. These researchers recommend briskly walking a total of three hours each week to beat pain, boost mood, and improve disability.

Only your doctor can help you decide which path to healing is right for you. Ask him to help you sort through the options and track your progress.

Smooth moves renew sore muscles

Stretches are gentle movements that will have your back feeling great in no time. They relax muscles, relieve pressure on your vertebrae, and lengthen your spine. The result – less stiffness and better range of motion.

- Lie on your back with both knees bent and your feet flat on the floor. Wrap your hands around one knee and gently pull it toward your chest. You'll feel a good stretch in your lower back. Hold the position for 20 seconds, release your knee, and repeat with the other leg.
- Stand up with your knees slightly bent and place your hands on the small of your back. Lean back and look at the ceiling. Hold for five seconds, then slowly straighten.
- While standing, take turns rolling each shoulder forward for 15 seconds, then backward. You can start with little circles and, as you gain flexibility, work your way up to larger ones.

With each exercise, you should feel a gentle stretch in your muscles. Stop immediately if there's any pain. And clear these stretches with your doctor before trying them, since they may not be right for you if you have certain types of back problems.

Water washes cramps away

Heal back pain with an everyday beverage? Sounds incredible, but simply drinking plenty of water can put an end to muscle cramps – one folk remedy that really does work.

Dehydration commonly causes muscle cramps, especially if you're working outdoors in the heat, exercising, or performing strenuous activities. Older folks are likely to suffer "heat cramps" partly because you lose some of your sense of thirst with age. Head these painful spasms off with advice from the American Academy of Orthopaedic Surgeons.

- Stop for water regularly, before you feel thirsty.
- Drink more than you need to quench your thirst.
- Consider fruit juices or sports drinks if you are working outside or sweating for more than an hour. They help replenish lost nutrients.

Good posture prevents injuries

Improve your posture and you've just taken the first – and the easiest – step to fewer back problems. So, take a load off your spine with this advice.

Stand up straight. Check your spine's alignment by standing with your heels against a wall. The back of your head, shoulders, buttocks, and calves should all touch the wall, and your hand should fit between the wall and the small of your back.

Not making the grade? Better straighten up. When you stand, stretch the top of your head toward the ceiling and relax your shoulders. Tuck in your chin and tighten your stomach muscles to better support your back. If you're standing for long periods, take turns resting one foot on a low stool to relieve pressure on your lower back.

Sit pretty. Look for a chair with low back support, and make sure your feet touch the ground. Your knees should be slightly higher than your hips. Prop them on a phone book or footstool if necessary. If sitting bothers your lower back, roll up a small towel to about the thickness of your forearm and sit with it behind the small of your back.

Music soothes savage aches

Backache have you snarling? Turn on some tunes. According to a French study, people with chronic low back pain who listened to music felt less depressed and anxious. And now new research from the Cleveland Clinic Foundation finds people with chronic pain who listen to tunes have less pain, depression, and disability. There's no scientific explanation for this, but experts say music could naturally boost the power of pain relievers. The kind of music doesn't seem to matter. So strike up the band, turn up the radio, or put on your old favorites – and take a musical interlude from pain.

Sleep habits: good nights mean better days

No more sleeping on a hard bed for back problems. A Spanish study found medium-firm mattresses did a better job relieving chronic low back pain than firmer ones. Not ready to splurge on a new bed? Slide a piece of plywood between a soft mattress and its box spring to firm it up. Try these other tips for more healing sleep.

- Lying on your back puts 55 pounds of pressure on your spine. If you tend to sleep in this position, tuck a pillow under your knees. This cuts the pressure in half.
- Slip a pillow between your bent knees if you like sleeping on your side – the best position for a bad back. This maintains the natural S-shaped curve of your spine and relieves pressure on it.
- Stop sleeping on your stomach. It puts unnecessary strain on your back and can prolong recovery from an injury.
- Give your back a hand getting up. Roll onto your side, swing your legs over the edge of the bed, and use one arm to push yourself to a sitting position.
- Avoid strenuous exercise first thing in the morning. Your spinal discs are full of fluid when you wake up, which makes them more prone to injury.

Vitamin D: a back-saving nutrient

Your aching back may just need a little tender loving D. Vitamin D deficiency can cause muscle weakness, osteoporosis, and unexplained aches and pains – and experts are shocked at how common it is. Out of 150 people who complained of general aches and pains

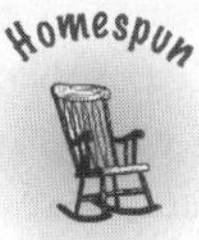

Mustard spreads muscle relief

Mustard lovers rejoice! A squirt of this saucy topping could spell relief from muscle cramps. Science doesn't prove it, but athletes swear by it. Some wash down a packet of mustard with water every two minutes until the cramp stops. Others say pickle juice does the trick. They down 2 ounces of pickle juice 10 minutes before game time to ward off cramps, and use the same remedy once a cramp takes hold.

in a recent study, 93 percent were vitamin D-deficient, and five had no vitamin D in their blood at all. Researchers were stunned.

This crucial nutrient helps you absorb calcium from food and supplements. Too little D means you absorb too little calcium. So, your body gets desperate and starts "stealing" calcium from your bones. Experts think weakened bones were behind the aches and pains in this study – and they could be causing yours.

Eating more foods fortified with vitamin D, like milk, can help you get back on track. But the best way to boost D levels is simply to spend a little time in the sun every day. You get up to 90 percent of your required vitamin D from sunlight. Just five to 15 minutes of sun on your face, hands, and arms without sunscreen, between 11 a.m. and 2 p.m. should do the trick. Talk to your doctor about safe ways of getting extra D if you have dark skin or live in a cold climate.

Super supplements stop the hurt

There's nothing fishy about these back pain remedies. Fish oil supplements and the herbs devil's claw and white willow bark may treat back pain as well as prescription drugs, but without risky side effects.

To prove this, experts isolated from fish oil two types of omega-3 essential fatty acids that specifically combat inflammation – eicosapentaenoic acid (EPA) and decosahexaenoic acid (DHA). They gave 1,200 milligrams (mg) every day to people with back and neck pain. After only about two months, nearly 60 percent were able to stop taking their prescription pain relievers. To get the same results, make sure your fish oil supplement contains EPA and DHA.

A separate review of 10 studies concluded both devil's claw (*Harpagophytum procumbens*) and white willow bark (*Salix alba*) relieve chronic low back pain, in some cases, as well as prescription pain relievers. Experts say these are safe for short-term treatment – four to six weeks – but need more research before recommending them long-term. For pain relief, buy a white willow bark extract that contains a daily dose of 240 mg of salicin, which acts much like aspirin in your body. Or try a devil's claw extract made with water, not ethanol, and containing 50 mg of harpagoside, a natural anti-inflammatory.

Hot peppers head off back pain

Rub out pain with a cool cream made from hot peppers. Some over-the-counter pain rubs, such as Zostrix, contain capsaicin, the compound that makes chili peppers so spicy hot. When you apply it to your skin, it excites nerve endings and triggers your body to release a chemical called "substance P" that carries pain messages to your brain. That's why your skin might burn, itch, or prickle when you first apply the cream. Over time, the capsaicin drains your body's store of substance P, which gradually deadens your sense of pain. You may get almost instant pain relief, or, like some people, you may need to rub it on several times a day for a week or two before your aches fade. Studies show capsaicin creams pack real relief from chronic muscle and joint aches, especially if you haven't had luck with other treatments. Just be sure to wash your hands after handling capsaicin.

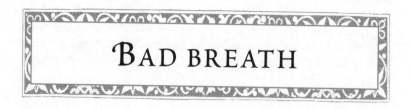

BAD BREATH

Banish bad breath with good habits

Everyone has unpleasant breath sometimes. When you first wake up in the morning or after you eat a garlicky meal, for instance. But some people have bad breath, also called halitosis, all the time. This can seriously hamper your social and professional life. Find out what causes bad breath and the simple steps you can take to prevent it.

Rule out the worst. Sometimes bad breath is a symptom of a more serious problem. Gum disease, digestive disorders, diabetes, liver or kidney failure, sinusitis, and respiratory infections may be to blame. Other possible causes include Sjogren's syndrome, vitamin deficiencies, and oral cancer. It may even be a psychological problem. Some people remain convinced they have bad breath, even when they don't. Treat these conditions, and you'll treat your halitosis.

Ace your oral exam. But in most cases, bad breath stems from bacteria in the mouth. These bacteria, which accumulate in hard-to-reach areas like the back of your tongue and between your teeth, produce foul-smelling substances called volatile sulfur compounds (VSCs). These gases give bad breath its odor. Practice good oral hygiene to get to the root of the problem.

- Brush at least twice a day and floss at least once. Make sure to brush your gums, cheeks, and roof of your mouth as well.
- Use a tongue scraper, spoon, or the bristles of your toothbrush to clean the back of your tongue, where bacteria lurk.
- Clean your dentures, bridges, and other dental appliances regularly.
- Go to the dentist twice a year for checkups.

- Drink plenty of water. When your mouth is dry, decaying food cells stick to your tongue and the inside of your cheeks, providing food for bacteria. Aim for at least six 8-ounce glasses a day.
- Breathe through your nose. When you breathe through your mouth, it can get dry.

Ruling out any serious conditions and improving your oral hygiene are the first steps in banishing bad breath. Read on for more helpful tips.

Freshness felons: what not to eat

Spit out that mouthwash. It may mask bad breath for a while, but if it contains alcohol it may do more harm than good. Alcohol can dry out your mouth, leaving it ripe for foul-smelling bacteria.

In addition, what you eat affects your breath – but for varying reasons. For example, when your body processes certain foods, it creates smelly chemical byproducts that move through your bloodstream

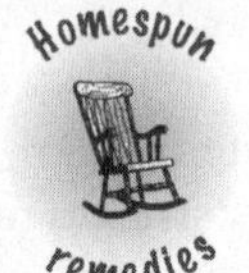

Chewable remedies freshen your mouth

Does your breath need a pick-me-up? Chew some sugarless gum to stimulate saliva production and wash away stinky bacteria. Or crunch on some high-fiber fruits and vegetables – like carrots, celery, and apples – to scrub pesky bacteria from the back of your tongue. You can also try chewing a variety of traditional folk remedies from around the world.

- parsley
- mint
- oregano
- dill
- fennel seeds
- anise seeds
- guava peels
- filberts
- cinnamon

and end up being exhaled through your lungs. Your bad breath won't truly go away until your body eliminates all the food. For this reason, if you're worried about bad breath, you should steer clear of these offending items:

- garlic
- onions
- pungent cheeses
- pastrami
- spicy foods
- fatty foods
- high-protein foods, like meat and eggs

Remember, protein and sugar provide fuel for the odor-causing bacteria in your mouth, and will send them into a growing frenzy. Tobacco products, coffee, and dairy tend to linger, creating distinctively bad breath. And you may not be able to avoid them, but certain medicines dry out your mouth, including antidepressants, antihistamines, decongestants, blood pressure drugs, anxiety drugs, and diuretics.

Yogurt creams bad breath

Dip your spoon into some yogurt, and dismiss bad breath. In a recent Japanese study, people who ate 6 ounces of sugar-free yogurt containing live active cultures each day for six weeks significantly reduced odor-causing compounds in their mouths. Researchers suspect the probiotics, or good bacteria, in yogurt counteract the bacteria that cause bad breath. In fact, probiotics are so promising that one company is developing a probiotic mouthwash. Although they work a bit differently, other foods can also freshen your mouth. Green, black, or white tea; cranberries; and wasabi – also known as Japanese horseradish – all contain antibacterial properties that may fight bad breath.

Bites & Stings

Tell backyard buddies to bug off

The National Insect Collection, maintained by the Smithsonian Institution, contains about 35 million bug specimens. That's a lot of creeping, crawling, flying critters. And since for every one of those unique specimens there's about a bazillion live ones out there that see you as either a threat or as food – or both – you're bound to get bitten or stung once in a while. It can feel like war, with the mosquitoes, ticks, bees, ants, hornets, spiders, and wasps winning. But while you may be outnumbered, you're not outgunned. There's help right at home for the pain or itch of many bites and stings.

Set mosquito bites to rights. You can blame the aggravation of a "skeeter" bite on one thing – mosquitoes are messy eaters. They leave a little of their saliva behind after biting. In fact, your body's defensive reaction to that saliva causes the itching, redness, and other symptoms. The next time a mosquito nips you, here's what to do.

☛ Wash the bite with soap and water.

☛ Don't scratch. Fingernails can spread infection.

☛ Use itch busters like calamine lotion, antihistamine creams like Benadryl, hydrocortisone creams, or the itch-fighting remedies in this chapter.

Watch out for sting operators. Wasps, hornets, yellow jackets, and fire ants can all sting, but only bees leave their stingers behind. Check for a black spot right where it hurts the most. If you find one, that's the stinger. Since it will keep pumping venom into your skin, try to remove it within the first minute. The stinger is barbed, so gently scrape it off with the edge of a credit card or some other clean flat object. Then wash the area with soap and water.

Your body will try to flush the venom out – that's why the wound swells and turns red. An ice pack can help control this, plus ease any pain. If you're still hurting, take an over-the-counter painkiller or use a pain-fighting remedy from this chapter. If you itch, use the same anti-itch strategies as you would for a mosquito bite.

Beware the web crawlers. Few spiders are truly dangerous – the black widow and brown recluse are two that are poisonous enough to be life threatening. You'll recognize the black widow by the red hourglass shape on its back, while the brown recluse sports a violin-shaped mark. Of course, you may never see the spider that bites you. For example, the first sign of a brown recluse bite may be a red mark that turns into a blister. You may start to feel feverish, nauseated, and develop a rash. A black widow's bite can cause muscle spasms, vomiting, cramps, and even partial paralysis.

Black widow

If you think you've been bitten by either of these pests, wash the bite area with soap and water, apply an ice pack, and get medical treatment right away.

Evict all ticks. These tiny parasites will come looking for you. So, check your body and clothes for ticks any time you go in woods, tall grass, or places where plants are thickly clustered. Because some may carry disease, you must quickly remove the tick, the whole tick, and nothing but the tick. If you leave some behind, contaminants could get into your bloodstream.

- Don't use bare fingers, nail polish, matches, or petroleum jelly. Instead, grab the tweezers. Position them against your skin so the tick is right between the two tines. Close the tines enough to grasp the tick but not enough to squeeze or flatten it.
- Pull upward slowly. You should see the skin pull and wrinkle slightly for several seconds before the tick lets go. Save the tick in a sealed baggie in the fridge.

Beware these deadly dangers

Call your doctor or 911 if you experience:

- rapid heartbeat; confusion; faintness; wheezing; difficulty breathing; loss of consciousness; rapid swelling where the sting or bite occurred; or swelling of the lips, tongue, or throat. Even if you have never had problems with bites or stings before, you could be having a life-threatening allergic reaction.
- fever, muscle aches, headache, a rash, swollen glands, shaking, or convulsions after a mosquito bite. These could indicate a case of West Nile virus.
- a rash or flu-like symptoms like headache, body aches, fever, neck stiffness, and chills. These can be signs of Lyme disease, transmitted by ticks.

- Wash the bite site and the tweezers with soap and water.
- Ask your local health department if you should test the tick.

3 best bite rescues

When nature attacks, look for relief in your pantry. Here are three simple remedies that are fast, cheap, and effective.

Aspirin. Soothe stings from bees, hornets, wasps, yellow jackets, or fire ants with this, but not the way you think. Sure, you can swallow one down and feel better, but there is a trickier way to benefit from aspirin's healing power. Find a bottle of aspirin – not the enteric-coated kind – and crush one tablet. Mix in just enough water to make a paste. Spread directly over the sting site, then cover with a bandage or first-aid tape so no aspirin oozes out. Doctors say it won't take long for this remedy to start fighting pain, swelling, and inflammation.

Baking soda. The acid in bee venom can keep burning long after you remove the stinger. Baking soda is alkaline, so it neutralizes this acid and puts out the fire. Pour some baking soda into your palm or a small saucer, and mix in just enough water to make a spreadable paste. Smooth this over your sting and leave it for at least 15 minutes. You can also use this remedy for other stings or to help stop itching from bug bites.

Meat tenderizer. First, check the label to make sure yours has the right ingredients. It can't have any added seasonings and must contain papain – a natural enzyme from papaya that helps break down venom. Only tenderizer that passes both tests will ease both itching and pain. To give your bite or sting "tender"izer loving care, mix the powder with water to make a paste. Then spread it over the area that is itching or hurting, and leave it on for up to 20 minutes.

Smart strategies help you beat the bugs

You can escape that next unpleasant insect encounter just by changing the way you dress and behave. Start fighting off mosquitoes with these tips.

- Avoid being outside during dusk and dawn. More mosquitoes are flying and biting during these times.
- Get rid of standing water in your yard. Mosquitoes breed and lay their eggs in it.
- Wear heavy long sleeves, long pants, and socks outdoors, since mosquitoes can bite right through thin fabric. If you must wear lightweight clothing, spray it – but not your skin – with an insect repellent containing DEET.
- Avoid alcohol. A small Japanese study discovered that more mosquitoes landed on people after they had drunk only 12 ounces of beer. The experts agreed the alcohol somehow attracted mosquitoes, but couldn't explain why. This phenomenon may also apply to other alcoholic drinks.

Here's how to protect yourself from stinging insects.

- Don't look or smell like a flower. That means no brightly colored clothing and a pass on perfumes; scented soaps, lotions, or hair products; and other fragrant cosmetics.
- Don't go barefoot outside, especially on flowering fields or clover-covered lawns.
- Swat not. Quick movements provoke bees, hornets, and wasps to sting. Just slip smoothly away from the buzz.
- Don't leave sweet food or sweet drinks uncovered or unattended outdoors. You could swallow a nasty surprise.

Beautyberry: a 'beaut' of a mosquito repellent

An old folk remedy from the Mississippi hills could lead to a new way to make pesky skeeters scatter. For years, people in the South have rubbed crushed leaves from the American beautyberry shrub (*Callicarpa americana*) on their skin to keep mosquitoes and other pests away.

Now, thanks to a botanist working for the U.S. Department of Agriculture, the American beautyberry may become even more famous. Charles T. Bryson learned of this remedy from his grandfather 40 years ago. At that time, the crushed leaves were used to keep biting insects from pestering draft animals, like horses and mules. Bryson and his colleagues decided to put the plant to the test – a lab

Homespun remedies

A little rub can wipe out bites

Check your medicine cabinet for just the thing to prevent mosquitoes from biting and stop the itch of existing bites. Grab your bottle of rubbing alcohol and splash a little on the bite to fight the itch. You might also send mosquitoes packing if you smooth rubbing alcohol on your skin and let it dry before you step outside.

test, that is. They isolated three compounds in American beautyberry leaves that repel mosquitoes. Future testing will determine whether these chemicals are safe and how long they keep working.

You may have a beautyberry growing in your yard right now – it's native to the southeastern United States. Look for a deciduous shrub sporting autumn and winter clusters of intensely purple berries close to its stems.

Ice that itch for relief

The itch is driving you nuts. But you know scratching that bite – especially with fingernails – is asking for trouble. Here's a way to scratch safely. Wrap a cloth or paper towel around one end of an ice cube and scratch with the other end. The ice is too smooth to damage your skin and the chill will freeze that itch.

New skeeter beaters shut down swatting season

Are you uncomfortable slathering on chemical repellents like DEET, but hate that you must reapply more natural products every hour or so just to keep them working? Science may have a better mosquito repellent – or two – just around the corner.

- You love what its minty-lemon flavor can do for a roast chicken. You'll love it even more when mosquitoes take one whiff of you and bite in the other direction. A Korean study found certain compounds in the perennial herb thyme repel mosquitoes better – and longer – than DEET.

- It drives your cats wild, but it also drives mosquitoes away. An essential oil in catnip proved 10 times more effective than DEET at repelling mosquitoes – at least in test tubes. Experts say the catnip compound may repel flies and cockroaches, too.

Of course, they'll do more testing – especially on human skin – before marketing these remedies as safe and convenient mosquito repellents, but stay tuned. Someday soon, you might be able to toss your DEET bottle and use these natural mosquito-busters instead.

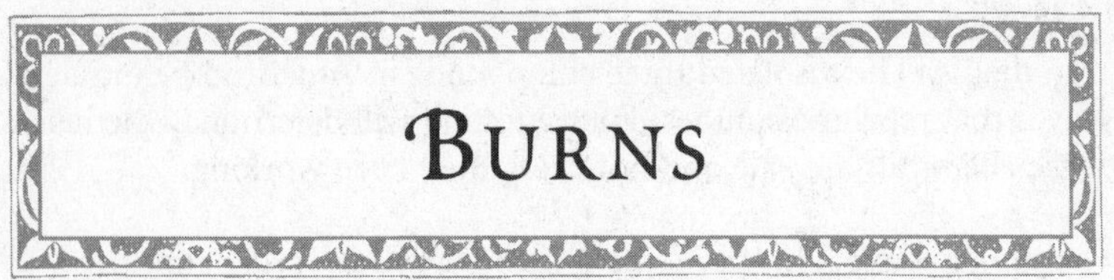

Burns

Fight the fire with first-rate first aid

What is tough, flexible, elastic, waterproof, and the largest organ in your body? Of course it's your skin. You may take for granted that it protects everything else in your body from things like germs, cold, sunlight, and heat – that is until you damage it. Then thank the millions of tiny nerve endings just under your skin for letting you know you've done something wrong. And nothing says "ouch" like a burn.

You can get burned by heat, chemicals, sunlight, or electricity. See a doctor immediately if your burn is larger than 2 inches, has fluid-filled blisters, or if your skin is charred and oozing. It's considered a first-degree burn, however, if cells only in the top layer of skin – the epidermis – are damaged. And you can treat a minor first-degree burn yourself. It may swell, turn pink or red, and perhaps whiten if touched briefly, but should never form blisters. Your goal is to prevent infection and let your body kick into its natural healing process. In no time at all, dead skin cells will slough off and new tissue will grow from the surrounding healthy skin.

Now in olden days, people used to blow on burns and say, "Blow in frost and come out fire." The blowing may make you feel a little better, but face it, it doesn't really matter what you say, you need to use some good commonsense emergency first aid:

- Cool the burn down with water.
- Clean it if needed.
- Cover it with antibiotic cream and gauze.

- Swallow an over-the counter pain reliever to ease the ache.
- Change the dressing regularly, keeping your scorched skin clean.

Remember, a sunburn is considered a first-degree burn. Check out the *Sunburn* chapter for some cooling, soothing remedies when you over-indulge.

Water first: perfect temp dampens pain

You can get instant pain relief if you use water the right way. Put your burned area under cool water immediately, but don't stop there. Soak the burn or keep it under cool, running water for 10 minutes. Cool water muffles the pain, reduces swelling, and lowers the temperature of your superheated skin. Just don't be tempted to use ice water or ice as a substitute. The drastic temperature difference between freezing ice and seared skin could make the damage worse.

Honey heals burns faster

It sounds like an old wives' tale, but experts are eager to dip into this particular honey pot – spread the sweet stuff over your burn and it just may heal faster. Research suggests that honey reduces the inflammation and pain of burns, speeds up healing, helps fight harmful bacteria, and encourages dead tissue to shed. In fact, burns covered with honey-saturated gauzes healed faster and with less infection than burns dressed with standard treatments.

Does this mean you can grab the jar out of your pantry and spread honey on your toast and your burn? Not quite. Store-bought honey is usually heat-treated and filtered, while many of the studies used raw honey. So what's the difference?

- Filtered honey means impurities have been removed and you're putting a more sterile product on your burn. This also means you shouldn't get toast crumbs in your first-aid honey.

- Heat-treating prevents honey from fermenting. But exposure to this kind of heat – as well as sunlight – diminishes honey's ability to fend off harmful germs.
- Raw honey is straight from the beekeeper's hives. That means it has never been heat-treated and impurities may not have been filtered out. You'll need to ask. To keep this kind of honey in top bacteria-fighting form, store it in a dark place that stays below 50 degrees Fahrenheit.

The bottom line is that store-bought honey may be less effective than raw honey that has been filtered. If you decide to try honey, remember to cool and clean the burn first, and keep the wound covered so it won't dry out.

Household plant holds amazing powers

Aloe vera has been called the burn plant, the medicine plant, and even the miracle plant. While there's not much hard clinical evidence to back up these names, aloe has been used as a healing remedy since ancient times. Many experts agree it has special ingredients that can treat wounds and inflamed skin.

Use aloe vera after you've cleaned and cooled a burn with water. Clip off a long leaf, wash it, and slit it open. Apply gel from the

MythBuster: Should you butter your burn?

Maybe you grew up thinking butter helps heal burns. But it simply traps heat in your skin – just like covering up a hot metal pot on a stove. The same is true for petroleum jelly. In fact, covering a burn in petroleum jelly can prevent it from healing and might even lead to infection, experts warn. Bypass these remedies so your scalded skin can cool.

inside of the leaf and cover your burn with a bandage. Change the bandage and the aloe at least once a day until the burn heals.

Be aware that you could experience an allergic reaction to aloe vera if you are allergic to garlic, onions, or tulips.

For potent and cheap aloe vera anytime, grow your own potted aloe on an indoor windowsill. The plant thrives on neglect and minimal watering.

Papaya: a traditional African remedy

Every day hospital staffers in the Republic of The Gambia in Western Africa mash fresh papaya to treat burn victims. It seems this regional folk medicine helps shed dead tissue and prevents infections. What's more, lab tests have shown that the papain enzyme in papaya may hasten burn healing. Just remember, if you are allergic to latex, you may also be allergic to papaya.

Antioxidants repair singed skin

Toss spinach leaves with fresh oranges, peach slices, strawberries, sunflower seeds, and almonds and you've got one delicious singe-soothing salad. These foods deliver plenty of the powerful antioxidants, vitamin C and vitamin E. That's good news because antioxidants defend your cells against the damaging free radicals burns unleash.

On top of that, a recent small study found that burn patients who took vitamin E and C supplements healed faster than patients who didn't. Although more research is needed, experts say scalds and burns can raise your body's need for antioxidant nutrients. So get plenty of vitamins E and C and see what their antioxidant power can do for you.

Cataracts

See your way to clearer vision

In 1922, cataracts forced the famous French artist, Claude Monet, to stop painting. He struggled with blurriness for years and nearly went blind before cataract surgery restored his sight. Fortunately, you can lower your risk of developing cataracts. Start by learning how cataracts develop.

Like the lens of a camera, your eye's lens focuses incoming light rays to create a distinct image. Your lens must remain clear for you to see well. In fact, your body has processes to help keep it that way. But growing older can change your body chemistry, causing proteins in your lens to clump together and form cloudy areas that can lead to cataracts. Cataracts cause the light rays to scatter – fogging over your vision like a pane of frosted glass.

So why doesn't everyone get cataracts as they grow older? Unstable molecules called free radicals may hold the answer. Your body naturally produces free radicals, but hazards like ultraviolet light from the sun and smoking can make your eyes produce too many. This overload of free radicals can trigger the changes in your eye's lens that eventually lead to cataracts.

Cataracts can take years to steal your vision, or they could erase it in just a few months. Once you have a cataract, surgery is your only hope of cure. You might prevent both the vision loss and the surgery if you take steps to avoid this common eye disease.

☛ Shed pounds if you're overweight.

- Eat foods rich in the antioxidant glutathione, which helps fight free radicals. Good choices include fresh asparagus, avocado, raw spinach, and potatoes.
- See your eye doctor for a regular checkup every year starting at age 60.
- Quit smoking. Smoking a pack, or more, of cigarettes a day nearly doubles your risk of developing cataracts.
- Avoid drinking alcoholic beverages. Drinking every day can raise your risk about 30 percent.
- Ask your doctor if you are taking medications that could raise your cataract odds. You might be able to switch to a drug with less risk.

Diabetes, eye injuries, and a family history of cataracts also increase your risk. If you get cataracts, you'll not only have to deal with dimmed or blurred vision, but also problems with night driving, double vision, sensitivity to glare, colors that appear muted, or poorer vision in bright light.

Tuna leads a school of sight defenders

Eating tuna to guard your eyesight may sound fishy, but you don't want to let this fish story get away. Cold water fish, like tuna, contain a powerful omega-3 fatty acid called docosahexaenoic acid (DHA), a nutrient that also naturally occurs in your eyes.

People with cataracts have less DHA in their eyes than people who don't have cataracts. That's why many scientists think DHA might fight cataract-causing changes in your eyes. In fact, a study of more than 70,000 women found that those who ate the most fish rich in omega-3s were less likely to get cataracts than those who ate the least fish.

But what about the claims that fish may be unsafe due to contaminants like mercury and polychlorinated biphenyls (PCBs). Fortunately, new reports from The Institute of Medicine and Harvard University

Beware diabetes eye dangers

People who have diabetes have a higher risk of glaucoma, diabetic retinopathy, and cataracts. Don't use home remedies for eye problems if you have diabetes. Get regular checkups from your eye doctor and see him immediately if you notice any changes in your eyes or vision.

say the benefits of eating fish outweigh the risks. These reports say most people can safely eat up to 12 ounces of store-bought fish weekly. Just make sure you eat more than one kind of fish if you have more than two servings a week. Good omega-3-rich choices include salmon, herring, sardines, and tuna. If you're planning meals for others, remember that children under age 12 and women who are pregnant or nursing should avoid shark, swordfish, tilefish, and king mackerel.

And there's more. A recent study found that eating too many landlubber fats, like corn oil, safflower oil, soybean oil, and sunflower oil might raise your odds of developing cataracts. Researchers say it might be a good idea to cut back on these fats, while adding fish to your diet.

Get the lead out for healthier eyes

Every time you drink a glass of tap water you could be raising your cataract risk. Many homes, especially those built before 1980, have hazardous lead in their water pipes or faucets, which can pass lead into the water you drink. New research shows exposure to lead can boost your cataract risk by interfering with the body processes that keep your eyes' lenses clear. Here are two ways you can protect your eyes from this hidden danger:

Install a water filter. Buy a water filter that claims on the package to remove lead from your water. As long as you can afford to change the replacement filters, this works well. If you don't change the filter regularly, it will stop removing lead.

Get your water tested. A two-sample water test can help you discover whether you can flush out accumulated lead simply by running the water from each tap for a few minutes every day.

The Center for Science and the Public Interest suggests you call your water authority or health department to ask about testing and prices. But, if that's too expensive, they also recommend a test kit from Clean Water Lead Testing, Inc., for under $30. To get prices and ordering information, call 828-251-6800 or write to Clean Water Lead Testing, Inc., UNCA, One University Heights, Asheville, NC 28804.

Plan to send two samples. Take the first one from the first run of tap water in the morning, before anyone showers or flushes. Take the second after the tap water has been running for about three minutes. If testing shows your second sample is lead free, you can let the water run for a few minutes every time you use each tap. Or do it once and fill up a few clean milk jugs with lead-free water for drinking and cooking.

Leafy greens to the rescue

Believe it or not, greens might be better for your eyes than carrots. Leafy greens contain two amazing phytonutrients – lutein and zeaxanthin – that are also found in your eyes' lenses. This dynamic duo ambushes harmful free radicals in your eyes. They may even help protect your lenses from damage by the sun's UV light. Best of all, you can easily get the lutein and zeaxanthin you need from foods – as long as you eat them with a little fat.

Start eating sunshine fresh greens like kale, collard greens, spinach, or Swiss chard. Surprisingly, you can also find some lutein and zeaxanthin in foods like celery, corn, tangerines, oranges, egg yolks, broccoli, kiwi, green peas, and honeydew melon.

Sunglasses: sunscreen for your eyes

Wearing sunglasses lowers your risk of developing cataracts. Out of 838 Chesapeake Bay fishermen, those who didn't wear sunglasses or wide-brimmed hats were three times more likely to get cataracts than those who did, researchers say. The invisible UV light in sunlight causes chemical reactions in your eyes that produce harmful free radicals. In fact, UV light can be so damaging even small amounts boost your cataract risk.

Sunglasses don't have to be expensive to offer maximum protection. Here are a few things to keep in mind.

- Read the label. It should say the sunglasses block 99 to 100 percent of ultraviolet (UV) light. Labels that say "block UV absorption up to 400nm," or those that feature the Skin Cancer Foundation's Seal of Recommendation for Sunglasses will give you the same mighty protection. But remember, don't settle for a label that only says "blocks UV." Know exactly what you're getting.
- Choose wraparound sunglasses with large lenses. Otherwise, UV light can creep in from the top and sides.

Many sunglasses offer lenses that are polarized, mirrored, or tinted a certain color, but none of these features block UV. Check the label to be sure you're getting maximum UV protection. Once you have good sunglasses, wear them anytime you're outdoors during daylight – even in the winter and on cloudy days. And don't forget to wear sunglasses when you drive. UV exposure is greater around pavement.

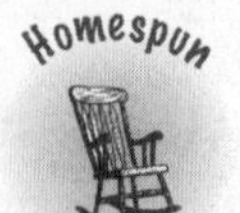

Mug cataracts with green tea

Green tea is chock-full of powerful antioxidants, and researchers think drinking it several times a day might slow down the development of cataracts. So far, it has only been tested in animals, but it's still worth a try. Besides, think how comforting a steaming mug of green tea can be.

COLDS & FLU

Simple steps help you survive sneeze season

You might think avoiding a cold or the flu is about as likely as dodging bullets in the OK Corral. Sure, colds are nothing to sneeze at – they prompt more doctor visits than any other condition. And the Centers for Disease Control and Prevention (CDC) says more than 200,000 people are hospitalized for the flu every year. But that doesn't mean you have to be a victim.

Colds and the flu are respiratory infections caused by viruses – tiny particles that lie around waiting for a host cell to infect. They get into your body through your nose, mouth, or broken skin and start wreaking havoc. Your immune system – a complex defense structure – kicks in and, if you're lucky, defeats the virus. If not, in two or three days, the virus will have reproduced and traveled throughout your body enough to start making you feel bad. You know the drill – sniffling, sneezing, coughing, headache, and sore throat.

If it's a cold, eventually, your immune system will win and you'll get better. That's why colds are called "self-limiting diseases." They run their course and go away. Hundreds of viruses can trigger a cold, but half of all colds come from the rhinovirus. Flu, which comes from the influenza virus, can sometimes be severe – with more uncomfortable symptoms than colds – or lead to pneumonia. If that's the case, your immune system could use some help. Antibiotics have no effect on a virus, but your doctor may prescribe drugs for flu complications. Your best move, of course, is to avoid colds and flu in the first place.

☛ Just by regularly washing your hands, you can banish viruses that cause colds, flu, even hepatitis A, plus many other serious ailments. This treatment takes only 10 seconds, costs less than 3 cents, and can be done anywhere there's clean water. Rediscover this traditional remedy, now proven by science. Don't be tempted by fancy antibacterial soaps – they don't offer special protection from viruses. Plain old soap and water work best.

- Try not to touch your face. Germs on your hands can easily enter your body through your eyes, nose, or mouth.
- Regular exercise keeps your immune system – and you – in good shape, by triggering the release of antibodies and "killer cells" that hunt down germs. Aim for 40 to 45 minutes of brisk walking each day.
- Avoid crowds and plane, bus, or train travel. The more people you are in close contact with, the greater your chances of picking up a bug.
- For people at high risk, including seniors, getting a flu shot before winter may be a good idea.

If you or someone in your household does get sick, make an effort not to spread germs. Sneeze or cough into a tissue, and throw it away immediately. Keep phones, doorknobs, remote controls, and other commonly touched areas in your home clean. And, of course, wash your hands frequently.

Lingering symptoms signal trouble

Just because you feel like you have a cold doesn't mean you have a cold. If symptoms persist for more than 10 days, see a doctor. You could have a more serious infection, like strep throat, sinusitis, or bronchitis. These require antibiotics or other prescription drugs to clear up.

In ancient times, you may have been advised to kiss a mule or rub yourself with goose grease to cure a cold. Even today, there's no shortage of bizarre advice, however, these are sound recommendations.

- Get lots of rest to give your immune system a chance to concentrate on fighting the virus.
- Drink plenty of liquids to keep your mucus thin and your body hydrated.

Here are some more good tips for preventing or dealing with colds and the flu.

Garlic: fight infections with flavor

Bad breath may be a small price to pay for good health. When you add garlic to your diet, you not only add great flavor – you also add protection from colds and flu.

Before modern antibiotics, garlic was used to treat outbreaks of dysentery, tuberculosis, and influenza. Today, you can still boost your immune system with this common pantry item. That's because garlic contains powerful sulfur compounds – including allicin – that fight infections by acting as natural antibiotics as strong as penicillin. In fact, garlic not only kills bacteria, but viruses and infectious fungi, too.

Raw garlic works best, but other forms can help – even supplements. A British study found that people who took one garlic capsule a day for 12 weeks had fewer colds and recovered faster from them than people who took a placebo.

Garlic is also a common ingredient in chicken soup, a longtime folk remedy that has been proven to ease cold and flu symptoms. So, eat more garlic. You might stay cold- and flu-free.

Spicy solutions for your symptoms

Over-the-counter cold medicines might relieve your symptoms, but they often leave you feeling dopey and drowsy. Luckily, you can find effective alternatives right in your spice rack. Here are some herbs and spices that do much more than just season your food.

Cayenne. This hot pepper makes your nose run and clears clogged sinuses, thanks to a substance called capsaicin. When you're stuffed up, a spicy meal may be just what the doctor ordered.

Horseradish. Like cayenne, horseradish can clear stuffy sinuses. Add a tablespoon of horseradish to a bit of honey. Both ingredients will kill bacteria, while the horseradish will break up mucus and force your sinuses open.

Turmeric. A staple of Indian cooking, this spice contains curcumin, which fights infections. Sprinkle turmeric in warm milk to soothe a sore throat.

Ginger. Clear your sinuses and fight infections with this root. You can also brew some soothing ginger tea or take ginger in capsule form.

Anise seed. This licorice-flavored herb acts as a natural antihistamine to dry up your runny nose.

Sage. You'd be wise to try this herb as a remedy for sore throats and coughs.

Lemon balm. Battle viruses with the leaves and stems of this lemony fresh herb.

Thyme. Make time for this herb with antibacterial properties to fight upper respiratory infections.

Just cooking with the right herbs and spices can help boost your immune system so you can fend off colds and flu. Your food will taste better, and you'll feel better.

Thyme

Sweet and sour combo soothes a cough

You never see Winnie the Pooh with a cough or a sore throat. That's no surprise, since the lovable cartoon bear is always eating honey. While it coats your throat to provide relief, honey also contains certain natural chemicals, called polyphenols, which have antioxidant and anti-inflammatory properties. As an antioxidant, honey fights bacteria, fungi, viruses, and cell damage. As an anti-inflammatory, it works to ease the swelling and pain in your body tissues. The darker the honey, the more powerful it is.

Combine honey with lemon, and you have a traditional – and effective – cold remedy. Lemon juice adds a punch of cold-fighting vitamin C and a splash of natural acid to battle bacteria. Just swallow a spoonful of the duo to soothe a sore, scratchy throat. Or sip a cup of hot tea with honey and lemon to relieve congestion and body aches. Get instant relief from a ticklish cough with an old-fashioned homemade cough syrup that actually tastes good. Simply drink warm lemon water with honey. Next time you get a cough or sore throat, reach for honey and lemon to make your symptoms more "bear-able."

Dissolve 2 aspirin in a glass of warm water to make a soothing sore throat gargle – just don't use coated or buffered aspirin. Or stir about ½ teaspoon of salt into 8 ounces of warm water. Experts say this gargle draws moisture out of the inflamed tissue in your throat, making it a bit easier to swallow.

New cautions for old standbys

Loading up on vitamin and mineral supplements to battle your cold may be a common strategy – but is it a wise one? Here's what you should know about some popular remedies.

Rethink zinc. This mineral plays a key role in maintaining your immune system, and a zinc deficiency can leave you vulnerable to infections. But that doesn't mean extra zinc is the answer. While some studies found zinc lozenges can shorten the life of a cold, just as many found no difference between zinc and a placebo. So the jury is still out on zinc as a cold remedy.

You may benefit from zinc, which is also available as a nasal spray or nasal gel, but at what cost? Too much zinc can lead to several problems, including constipation, nausea, copper deficiency, and mouth irritation from the lozenges. High doses of zinc may even increase a man's risk for prostate cancer.

Don't count on C. Long touted as a cold remedy, supplemental vitamin C may not be as powerful as once believed. Recent research shows that it does not prevent or cure colds – but with it, you may not feel quite so bad, for quite as long. One review found vitamin C supplements only helped people exposed to extreme cold or physical exertion, like skiers or marathon runners. High doses of vitamin C come with risks of headaches, kidney stones, and intestinal problems. It can also interfere with some medications and treatments.

MythBuster: Can a wet head cause a cold?

Your mother probably warned you not to leave the house with a wet head, or you'd catch a cold. While chances are greater you'll fall victim to one in the winter, experts say it has more to do with spending time indoors, where germs are plentiful, than with the temperature. Still, drying your hair and bundling up can't hurt since researchers are looking into the theory that cold temperatures constrict blood vessels, slowing the arrival of germ-fighting white blood cells. In other words, wet hair won't make you catch a cold, but you might be more susceptible to one if you get chilled. I guess your mother might be right after all.

Inquire about E. There's some good news here. One study found nursing home residents who took 200 international units (IU) of vitamin E each day had fewer colds during the course of a year. But other research had less rosy results. In fact, according to a review of 19 studies involving 136,000 people, higher doses of vitamin E can boost your risk of heart failure and cancer.

Your best bet is to get your vitamins and minerals from foods – not from supplements. A healthy, balanced diet does wonders for your immune system. Good food sources of vitamin C include oranges and other citrus fruits and juices, strawberries, broccoli, and dark leafy greens. You can find vitamin E in vegetable oils, nuts, seeds, and wheat germ, while meats, shellfish, legumes, and whole grains contain zinc.

Healing herbs: mixed bag of cold relief

Echinacea is such a popular herbal remedy for colds and flu that it literally flies off the shelves – to the tune of more than $300 million a year – but it doesn't exactly pass scientific tests with flying colors. And, as you can see, even some of the experts disagree.

- The National Center for Complementary and Alternative Medicine says there's no evidence echinacea prevents colds or flu – nor does it shorten their course.
- Stanford University School of Medicine reviewed several positive echinacea studies and found most had some sort of fatal flaw, such as an obvious difference between the herb and the placebo.
- The Center for Complementary Medicine Research, Technical University of Munich says echinacea may help you get over a cold faster, but won't prevent it in the first place.

Yet, some experts remain convinced of its power. They find fault with negative studies for using the wrong preparation or dosage of echinacea, or testing it among the wrong subject groups. If you decide to give echinacea a try, aim for a total daily dose of 500 to 1000 milligrams in capsule form, three times a day for up to a week.

But echinacea is not your only option. Here are some other herbal remedies that may help fight colds and flu. Just remember, because supplements are not regulated in the United States, you can never be completely sure of what you are taking.

Elderberry. You'll find this antiviral herb in the liquid supplement Sambucol. Two studies, one conducted in Norway and the other in Israel, found that Sambucol helped flu patients improve about twice as fast as those taking a placebo.

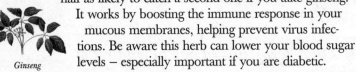

Ginseng. This ancient Chinese remedy might keep you from getting multiple colds. While you can still catch one cold, you are only about half as likely to catch a second one if you take ginseng. It works by boosting the immune response in your mucous membranes, helping prevent virus infections. Be aware this herb can lower your blood sugar levels – especially important if you are diabetic.

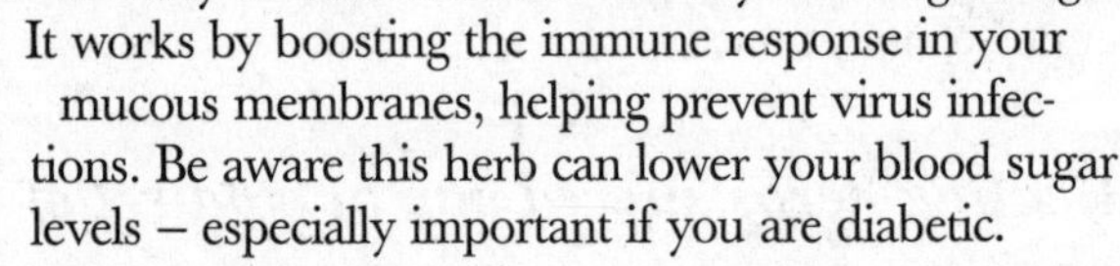

Ginseng

Cherry bark. Available as a tea or tincture, wild cherry bark may wallop your dry, hacking cough. There's no scientific evidence, but in the early 1900s, most cough syrup came from the bark of the wild cherry tree.

Goldenseal. Some believe this herb boosts the effects of echinacea, so you'll often find these combined in cold products.

Probiotics offer infection protection

There's a constant battle going on within your body. Harmful bacteria duke it out with the "good" kind that protect you. These good bacteria, also called probiotics, can help ward off many health problems, including respiratory infections. Here are some encouraging results from recent clinical research.

- People who drank milk fermented with the probiotic *Lactobacillus casei* cut the length of their respiratory infections by 20 percent.

- Workers needed fewer sick days when they had a daily dose of the good bacteria *Lactobacillus reuteri.*

- A probiotic "cocktail" every day can reduce the amount of harmful bacteria in your nasal passage.
- You can perk up your immune system with a regular measure of probiotics.

You've got nothing to lose and a whole lot of infection protection to gain by adding probiotics to your daily routine. You'll find them in fermented milk products and in yogurt – just look for "live active cultures" on the label.

Humidifier hygiene helps your health

Dry winter air can wreak havoc with your nasal passages, leaving you ripe for sickness. A humidifier might be the solution, but if you don't keep it clean, it will do more harm than good – and you'll end up with a breeding ground for mold, fungi, and bacteria.

- Choose distilled water over tap water, if possible. It doesn't contain minerals that feed bacteria.
- Change the water every day. This keeps deposits from building up inside.
- Clean the humidifier every three days. Chlorine bleach, a 3 percent hydrogen peroxide solution, or one-fourth cup of vinegar will do the trick. Check the instructions that came with your unit before cleaning, and rinse the tank thoroughly after cleaning with any chemical.
- Change the filter regularly.
- Check the humidity setting. It should be between 30 percent and 50 percent. Anything higher encourages bacteria, mold, and fungi.

CONSTIPATION

Gentle ways to get a move on

Did you cringe when Aunt Polly gave Tom a dose of castor oil in *The Adventures of Tom Sawyer*? Then you may be old enough to recall this traditional remedy for constipation. As bad as it tastes, this one works – and so do many other folk treatments like senna tea, honey, and flaxseed. While some remedies are gentle, others are downright potent, so make sure the cure fits the disease before you try a dose.

The good news is you can treat and even prevent colon slowdown by following some simple lifestyle rules.

- Go with the urge. The longer stool remains in your large intestine, the more water is drawn out. The result is hard, dry stool that's difficult to pass.
- Don't force it. Straining during bowel movements can cause tearing or hemorrhoids.
- Get some exercise. If you are older or don't move around much, you can really benefit from upping your daily physical activity.
- Check your medicines. Some drugs like narcotic painkillers, diuretics, antidepressants, iron supplements, and antacids with aluminum can stop things up.

It's better if you can get things moving without harsh laxatives, since they can be hard on your system and may be habit-forming.

Old standbys work best in combination

First things first. Before you try strong chemicals or quackish-sounding cures to bring on nature's call, try adding more fiber and water to your diet.

Make friends with fiber. Most Americans eat only 5 to 20 grams of fiber each day, while the American Dietetic Association suggests up to 30 grams for people over 50. That counts both soluble fiber, which feeds intestinal bacteria to increase stool mass, and insoluble fiber, which stays as roughage to help move food along and increase the volume of stool. You can get fiber from certain foods or from natural bulk-forming laxatives like psyllium or flaxseed. If that doesn't sell you on fiber's goodness, know this – along with battling constipation, getting the right amount of fiber every day can help fight off heart disease, stroke, and diabetes.

- Do it with diet. Whole grains, bran, beans, vegetables, and fresh fruits are great sources of fiber, while meat and dairy products are not. If you've been shying away from these fiber-filled foods, add them to your diet gradually to avoid problems with gas.
- Try some psyllium. Seeds of the psyllium plant are the basis of some common laxatives like Metamucil and Fiberall. Psyllium

MythBuster: Is daily go a must?

Don't believe the adage that nature should call every day. It's normal and healthy to have bowel movements less often – from three times a day to three times a week. Instead of worrying about strict regularity, pay attention to changes – in how often you go or what your bowel movements look like. If stool is hard and shaped like small pellets and this change lasts more than a week, you might have a problem.

works in two ways – it has lots of fiber and the seed coat is made of about 30 percent mucilage. This gooey stuff holds water in the stool, keeping it lubricated and moving. Try a teaspoon of psyllium seeds mixed with water at each meal, or follow the directions on the label of a psyllium product.

- Find relief in flaxseed. The seed – but not the oil – bulks up your stool. It also encourages your digestive muscles to contract and relax, forcing the contents of your intestines onward. You can take two to three tablespoons of flaxseeds stirred into a large glass of water.

Mix fiber with water. Drinking water every day is important for anybody with constipation, but if you increase your fiber, more water is critical. Without enough, all that fiber acts like a logjam in your intestines. Water washes through, softening your stool and keeping things lubricated enough to move along. In fact, studies show that the combination of fiber and water is the best way to get real constipation relief without using laxatives. Experts say to drink eight to 10 glasses of water daily.

Fabulous fruits are all-star fare

Many great-tasting fruits and vegetables are high in fiber, making them ideal weapons in the battle against constipation. Even better, certain fruits offer added benefits that help keep you regular. Don't waste money at the drugstore when these foods can do the trick.

Concentrate on kiwi. Rumor has it this luscious fruit from Down Under is great for constipation. Sure, it's chock-full of vitamin C and boasts almost 3 grams of fiber in each piece, but what about scientific proof? Well, researchers in New Zealand have it. They studied healthy seniors who added two to three kiwis to their usual daily diets. Overall, most people reported more frequent, easier bowel movements while on the kiwi diet. Researchers think that, along with the fiber, kiwi's cell walls hold extra water, adding to its laxative effect.

Plan on a papaya. Its rich orange color is a clue that the papaya is high in vitamin A. In addition, one piece of fruit contains more than 5 grams of fiber plus certain enzymes – including papain, which helps digest proteins. Papain works so well it's used to make digestive enzyme supplements.

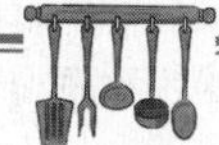

Try a rise-and-shine smoothie with fruit and fiber – a great combination to help move things along. In a blender, mix 1 cup of chopped fruit with:

- 1 tablespoon of psyllium (Metamucil) *or*
- 1 tablespoon of flaxseed *or*
- 3 tablespoons of rice bran

Add 8 ounces of water or fruit juice. You may want to avoid using bananas, which some people find constipating.

Indulge in figs. Need an excuse to eat fig bars – how about extra fiber? Two dried figs provide more than you'll find in one apple or five dates, and as much as you'd get in one half-cup of dried plums. All this concentrated fiber helps bulk up stool to really move your bowels along.

Honey gets nod from science

"Eat honey, my son, for it is good," was King Solomon's advice thousands of years ago. (Proverbs 24:13) Indeed, drinking one to three spoonfuls of honey in a glass of warm water is an age-old folk remedy for constipation. And this one really works.

Honey's sweetness comes from a mix of sugars – fructose, glucose, and sucrose. The exact blend is different depending on where the honey is produced and what kinds of flowers the honeybees find, but all honey has more fructose than glucose. Experts say the extra fructose doesn't digest completely, and this causes stool to move more quickly through your bowels.

To test the ancient remedy of honey for constipation, researchers asked some healthy people to drink honey in water and others to drink various mixtures of the sugars. Those who drank the honey mixture had softened stools, while the other group did not. Sounds like some great-tasting relief.

Fennel: tiny seed with stimulating powers

You may have seen a dish of fennel seeds offered as an after-dinner treat at Indian restaurants. These tiny tidbits do more than spice your mouth with a licorice-like taste, they also aid digestion by boosting your body's production of certain digestive enzymes and then helping them work better. Studies show fennel ups intestinal movement to shorten food transit time. This means it takes food less time to move all the way through your digestive system. And that means you move your bowels more often for constipation relief.

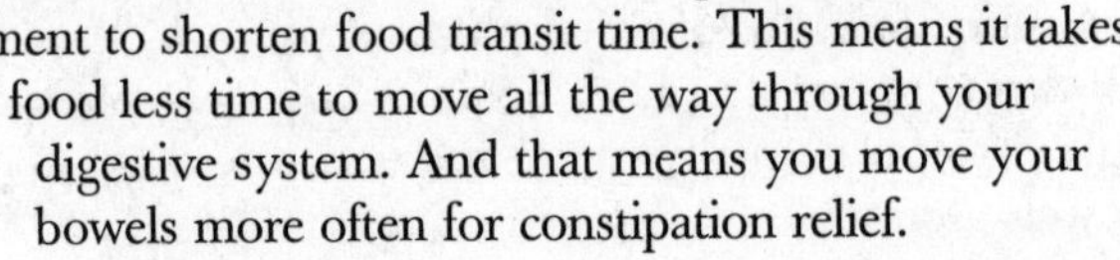

Fennel

This has other benefits, too. The less time waste spends in your colon, the lower your risk of colon cancer from toxins trapped there. In addition, drinking fennel tea or chewing fennel seeds releases a natural chemical called anethole, which blocks the series of steps that leads to cancer cell growth.

See the chapters on *Gas*, *Heartburn*, and *Irritable bowel syndrome* for more on fennel's powers to heal other ills, including diarrhea, stomachaches, indigestion, and cramps.

Tasty brews can help you go

Some plants and herbs offer constipation relief by acting as stimulant laxatives. Unlike fiber, considered a bulk laxative because it bulks up and softens your stool, these remedies encourage the smooth muscles of your intestines to get to work. The effect is usually quick, often shorter than two hours, and more powerful than with bulk laxatives.

Drugs like Correctol and Dulcolax work as stimulant laxatives, but you may prefer to go straight to the plant for speedy results. Try brewing up one of these get-moving remedies. Cascara sagrada and senna are available as teas and capsules in herb shops and health food stores. Coffee – well, you probably already have a pot brewing in your kitchen.

Cascara sagrada, or "sacred bark," is the aged bark of the buckthorn tree. It contains natural chemicals called anthraglycosides that cause more water and electrolytes to pass into the stool in your intestines. This bulkier, softer stool triggers muscle contractions that move things along faster.

Senna works by causing rhythmic muscle contractions in your intestines that move stool, and by encouraging more fluid to pass into your gut. Both cascara sagrada and senna can cause your urine to appear brownish, but this effect is harmless.

Coffee is a favorite morning pick-me-up that stimulates your brain, but it also stimulates your intestines to get in motion. Be aware, however, that the caffeine in coffee, tea, and other drinks tends to flush water from your body through your kidneys. This can bring on dehydration and trigger even worse constipation.

Experts say stimulant laxatives, whether herbal or more traditional over-the-counter products, are for occasional use only. If you take them too often, your body "forgets" how to operate without them.

M-o-M overload can spell danger

Laxatives like milk of magnesia are made of magnesium hydroxide. Too much can make you feel dizzy, confused, weak, and sick to your stomach. Call your doctor if you develop these problems while taking a magnesium-based laxative. If you have kidney problems, don't take milk of magnesia at all.

You can even permanently damage your intestine and colon. Talk to your doctor if you develop unusual symptoms.

Belly rub may get bowels moving

Try treating your constipation from the outside in – especially if internal remedies don't do the trick. A review of research in England found abdominal massage therapy to be of real help. Here's how to give yourself this kind of rubdown and help get your bowels going again.

Lie on your back with your knees bent and your feet flat on the floor but close to your body. Take a deep breath, letting the air fill your abdomen like a big balloon. Then let your breath out, pulling in your belly. Repeat this breathing pattern two more times. Hold your hands in gentle fists and begin rubbing your belly in small circles. Work in a clockwise pattern, the same direction your bowels flow. Go up the right side of your body, across under your ribs, then down the left side. Repeat up to 10 times, then finish with some more deep breaths.

Aloe juice can clear up constipation

Aloe juice, made from the skin of aloe leaves, is an ancient cure for constipation. It contains natural compounds called aloins, which bacteria in your colon breaks down in order to stimulate your digestive tract. When that happens, stool moves more quickly through your intestines. There's less time for your body to draw water out of the stool. And more water in the stool makes it softer, easing constipation.

You can buy aloe supplements in capsule or liquid form at drugstores or health food stores. Don't take more than directed on the package, or you may turn your constipation into diarrhea. It's also possible to become dependent on aloe juice, so you shouldn't take it for more than two weeks.

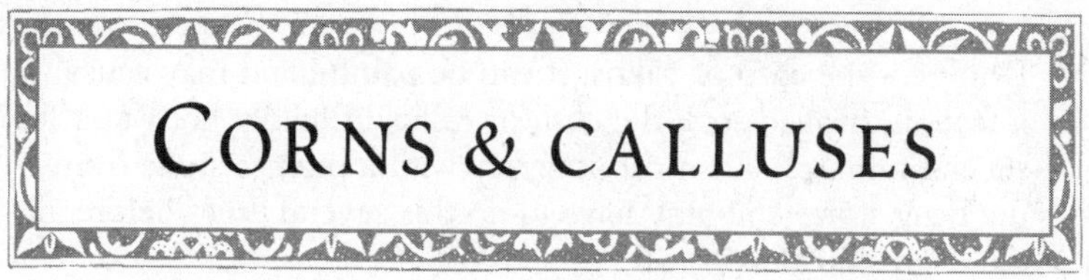

Corns & Calluses

Smart solutions to stop the pain

Corns and calluses can turn stepping out into an ouch at every step. These painful patches spring from several uncomfortable causes, but shoes are the most notorious offender.

That's because high heels, tight shoes, and other ill-fitting footwear can scuff against part of your foot or even bear down on it. Flawed shoes can also make your toes chafe against each other. That's definitely a case of getting off on the wrong foot, and here's why.

Continued friction or pressure on your foot makes the irritated area build up a hard core of dead skin. If the rough spot is on the soles of your feet, it's called a callus. But if it's on your toes, you have a corn. You can even get a "soft corn" between your toes, so named because moisture there keeps it from hardening.

Fortunately, home treatments can help most people. Use these tips to help save your soles – and your toes – so you can put your best foot forward again.

- Avoid socks that are too tight around your foot. Instead choose thick socks to limit chafing.
- If you spend long minutes standing at the kitchen sink, the stove, or the bathroom mirror, invest in a soft rubber mat to buffer your feet from the hard floor.
- Cushion your feet with insoles, corn or callus pads, or toe padding as needed.

- Don't cut the corn or callus. It can be painful and may cause infection. Instead soak the corn or callus in mildly hot water for several minutes. Then rub it gently with a pumice stone from the drug store. You may have to do this several times before all the dead skin sloughs off.

And remember, home treatments are not for everyone. If you have diabetes or poor circulation, skip the home remedies and see your doctor.

Lamb's wool cushions tender spots

You could tuck cotton or lamb's wool between your toes to help prevent corns or to ease the pain if you already have them. But any time you have a choice, pick lamb's wool. It won't compress into a useless wad or hang on to moisture like cotton does. Ask about lamb's wool padding at your favorite drugstore.

Lemon: skin softener with a-peel

You can sleep off a corn if you have a fresh lemon in the fridge. Just tape a bit of lemon peel to your corn. Then let it do the work while you catch some Z's. The citric acid in lemons can soften and exfoliate skin. What's more, if the corn is still tender, you can try swabbing the area with fresh lemon juice. Just be sure to let it dry before you cover your feet or walk around.

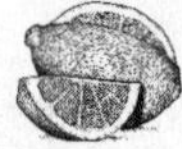

Petroleum jelly curbs calluses

Soften up hard corns and calluses with good old-fashioned petroleum jelly. If you're out of petroleum jelly, try lanolin hand cream.

Top tips for a good shoe fit

Throw your poor "dogs" a bone. Give them the best-fitting shoes you can find so corns and calluses become a thing of the past. Here's how.

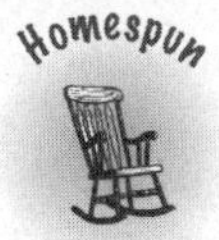

Easy Amish poultice banishes corn

According to the Amish, this old remedy makes corns vanish. Create a vinegar poultice and bind it to the corn. And don't worry about this poultice being messy or complicated to make. A slice of vinegar-soaked bread could be all you need.

- Shop late in the day so you won't buy shoes that are too tight. Doctors say your feet naturally swell as the day goes on.
- If you regularly wear inserts, insoles, or pads in your shoes, take them with you when you shop. Wear them when you try on new shoes.
- Try on both shoes in a pair. Walk around in them to be positive they fit comfortably. And don't settle for shoes that feel like they need "breaking in."
- Check for slippage. Shoes that are too loose can cause calluses and corns because your foot slides around too much.
- One foot can be just slightly larger than the other. Buy the size of shoe that fits that foot.
- Don't choose a shoe on the size number alone. Experiment with slightly bigger and smaller sizes than your usual. Check narrower and wider widths, too. That way you'll get footwear that's truly comfortable.
- Don't settle for less than a half-inch of space between the end of your longest toe and the toe end of the shoe.
- Be sure the widest part of the shoe is near the ball of your foot.
- Check that the heel fits snugly and comfortably.

- If you must wear high heels, choose shoes with plenty of toe room, cushioned insoles, and wide heels. Wear them as little as possible.

Salicylic acid: handle with care

Aspirin and corn treatments have something in common. Their active ingredient is salicylic acid, a medicine that comes from willow bark. Many ointments and medicated pads use this acid to remove corns and calluses. But take great care if you try them – doctors say salicylic acid could cause infections or even burns. If a skin or foot product with this ingredient has ever irritated your skin, ask your doctor or pharmacist about acid-free ointments for corns and calluses. And avoid foot products with salicylic acid if you have diabetes or poor circulation.

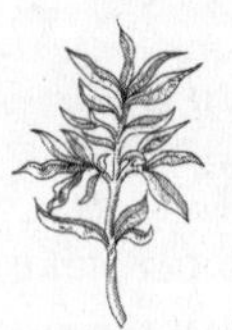

Willow

Pad your vacation against pain

It's day two of your dream vacation, and you're getting corns from the new shoes you bought for the trip. But you can help ease the pain and prevent new corns and calluses. Just learn how to pick the proper pads.

Pads can stop the rubbing and pressure that causes corns and calluses. So head for the foot section of a local drug store, and look for unmedicated pads. You can choose toe sleeves, gel cushions, insoles, or donuts. Pick toe sleeves to help corns between your toes. Try insoles and cushions to pad other parts of your feet.

But if you already have a corn, nab a doughnut-shaped pad. Corns have a hard, pointy core that aims inward. That means the core may press on a nerve every time you take a step. Surrounding the core with a doughnut takes the pressure off so the pain just goes away.

Cuts & Scrapes

Wise ways can 'make it better'

Your body's amazing healing process kicks in before you can even squeeze a tear out over your latest nick or scratch. The trick is to let this process take its course as naturally as possible. Unfortunately, through the ages, man has interfered in all kinds of strange and unusual ways. Tobacco, soot, spider webs, and various animal parts are all part of healing folklore. Every sort of leaf and root has been made into a poultice or bandage, some more successfully than others. And who could stock a first-aid kit without ointment of dragon? But not all remedies are so far-fetched. Even scientists are finding promise in some old cures for minor cuts and scrapes.

Boost home healing. Some remedies work best right after you've injured yourself, while others work better if you use them a few hours or days later. Learn your body's four steps of healing so you'll apply the right remedy at the right time.

- When you get a paper cut or skin a knee, your body's emergency responders spring into action. First, your blood vessels constrict temporarily so you lose less blood. Then, like an ambulance full of paramedics, clotting agents rush in to place a temporary seal over the damage.
- Inflammation sets in next, causing redness, swelling, and pain. But the good news is that it also relaxes your blood vessels so helpful white blood cells can flood your damaged tissues. They storm in, clean out dead tissue and dirt, and destroy infection-causing bacteria. White blood cells usually stop converging on the injured area after a few days. Yet if you aren't getting the right nutrients, inflammation could continue longer than it should.

- Just as construction crews craft frames for buildings out of wood or steel, a group of cells called fibroblasts build a framework for skin from substances like protein and collagen. In the next few days to weeks, new skin cells spread across the framework, until the wound closes.

- In the months that follow, collagen helps build new tissue until the skin is almost as strong and healthy as it was before you got hurt.

Now that you know what happens when you heal, you'll be more likely to use each remedy when you need it most.

Manage the damage. Some cuts and abrasions are so tricky or severe they can't be treated with just home remedies and first aid. See a doctor if any of these apply to you.

- You can't clean the wound.
- You can't stop the bleeding.
- You haven't had a tetanus shot in the last 10 years.
- The wound is ragged or wide open.
- You're running a fever of more than 100 degrees Fahrenheit.

Fortunately, you can usually treat minor cuts and scrapes at home. Learn these vital steps to wound care first so you know when to include the home remedies you'll soon read about.

- Rinse with tap water or a sterile saline solution. Then wash the skin around your wound with a clean, soapy cloth and water. Pat dry with a cloth or paper towel.

- Press with a sterile bandage to stop the bleeding. If you are still bleeding after 10 minutes, see a doctor.

- Apply your choice of healing ointment like an antibiotic cream or honey. Cover with a bandage.

- Change the dressing regularly and keep the wound clean.

- See your doctor if the cut becomes more painful or more red, begins to swell, won't close, or leaks fluid that's thick, yellow, or green.
- If you can exercise without damaging the wound, go ahead. A small study of older adults, suggests regular exercise could speed up healing by as much as 25 percent.

Next you'll find some promising remedies that might help heal your cuts and scrapes. Just remember, if you have diabetes, check with your doctor before trying them.

Honey: sweet treatment fights infection

You may not need expensive ointments for that cut or scrape. Many kinds of honey act as a natural antibiotic, battling infection and healing minor wounds. Of course, scientists say they still need more evidence before they can clear honey for widespread use. But, if the early studies are right, this sweet golden liquid delivers healing effects like these:

- fights infection by drawing life-giving moisture away from bacteria
- helps reduce inflammation
- produces just enough hydrogen peroxide to act as a mild antiseptic but not enough to kill your cells

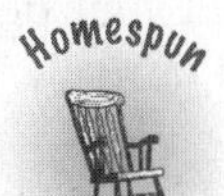

Wound cleaning made easy

Don't let an open wound get crusty and infected. Help it keep healing with a gentle antiseptic rinse. Measure out 2 cups of water. Then grab your measuring spoons and mix in 1 teaspoon of white vinegar. Use this tonic to rinse the wound and wash old, dead tissue away whenever you change the bandage.

- draws fluid from the wound to help the damaged area clean itself out
- may lessen scarring

You may choose to apply honey during the first-aid step instead of an antibiotic ointment. But remember the honey you buy in the grocery store may not help minor wounds resist infection. See the *Burns* chapter to learn how to choose and use a more powerful honey.

Meanwhile, if you don't have the right honey, make a sugar paste. Like honey, sugar pulls water from a wound – that may shut down infecting bacteria and help the wound shed dirt and other troublemakers. It may even help prevent scarring.

Make this homespun remedy with plain old granulated table sugar and just enough water to form a paste. Remember, sugar can affect your blood's ability to clot, so wait until one day after the bleeding stops before trying sugar paste.

Nutrients jump-start healing

A scrumptious roast turkey sandwich with a glass of orange juice could put a slow-healing wound back on the road to recovery. That's because these foods contain three must-have nutrients for damage repair – vitamin C, protein, and zinc. Doctors say deficiencies in these nutrients may be more widespread than previously thought. So, if you have wounds that mend sluggishly, tell your doctor about it and ask if you could be deficient. Here's why it matters and what you can do to help yourself.

Vitamin C helps make the collagen your body uses to rebuild damaged tissue. Yet, vitamin C deficiency is common in older adults and milder shortages occur in all ages. To make sure you get enough, enjoy more foods like sweet peppers, orange juice, cranberry juice cocktail, peaches, strawberries, and papaya.

Guard against allergic reactions

Allergies aren't just about sneezing. If you're allergic to something, rubbing it on your skin could give you a rash. So, start small when you try a new remedy. The American Academy of Dermatology says to test it out by applying a tiny bit to healthy skin, holding it in place with tape for a few days. If redness, itching, or other problems develop, don't use it – on wounds or on undamaged skin.

Zinc is a necessary mineral for several healing processes. But if you take certain medicines for high blood pressure like captopril (Capoten or Capozide), drugs that reduce stomach acid, or thiazide diuretics, your body may absorb less zinc than you think. Rack up more of this mending mineral with Total or Product 19 cereals, baked beans, lean ground beef, and turkey.

Proteins are key building blocks for restoring damaged skin and preventing inflammation from sticking around too long. In fact, without enough protein in your bloodstream, experts say you may take significantly longer to heal. Include high-protein foods such as chicken, turkey, fish, and lean meats in your diet or try protein-packed vegetarian combos. Pick from bean and rice dishes, pasta with cheese, black-eyed peas with rice, or even a cheese sandwich.

Sunscreen stands firm against scars

Your wound is healing and now you see the fresh pink of new skin. Before you go for a day of fun in the sun, grab the sunscreen. Your new skin will be super sensitive for several months and could still scar if it gets too much exposure to sunlight.

MythBuster: Best way to disinfect?

You don't need those stinging solutions from your childhood to disinfect cuts and scrapes. Today's doctors are holding up a big red stop sign for some drugstore disinfectants – including rubbing alcohol, hydrogen peroxide, and iodine-based products like Betadine. They've discovered these can be strong enough to damage your skin and even slow its healing. Their recommendation? Stick with good old soap and water.

Liquid bandage beats super glue

The next time you have a paper cut, don't be so quick to reach for that over-the-counter, household super glue. Note the warning on most labels: "avoid contact with skin." That's because they can irritate your skin and may even cause allergic reactions. In fact, if you use this glue on large wounds, it could produce enough heat to cause skin burns. But there's even more. If you don't seal your wound properly, the only way to remove the glue is with nail polish remover. Not only is that painful, but it can aggravate your poor damaged skin.

Fortunately, Band-Aid brand Liquid Bandage can do the job of super glues without the dangers or the damage. The makers of Liquid Bandage promise it won't sting or irritate, and because it's sterile, it's safer and better for you than super glues. They also say it's especially good for friction blisters, hangnails, paper cuts, and finger cracks. Plus you can easily remove it with baby oil or mineral oil.

In this case, it's better for your health and safety to pick a product designed specifically for the job at hand.

Vitamin E: no help for scars

Vitamin E may be famed as a top antioxidant for skin, but the latest research suggests you won't prevent or reduce scarring if you squeeze a vitamin E capsule or rub vitamin E cream on a wound. In fact, one study shows you're more likely to see one of these results:

- Your skin flares up with an allergic reaction.
- Your scar gets worse.
- Your scar shows no improvement.

Researchers continue to investigate, so stay tuned. But before you try vitamin E on your wounded skin, talk to your doctor.

Handy glove trick halts hand infections

Hand bandages are nearly impossible to keep clean and firmly attached, but now you can do it with ease. To protect dressings on your palm, knuckles, or the back of your hand, cut the fingers out of a snug-fitting latex glove and wear it when you need to do soggy or grubby work. Your bandage should stay clean and dry, cutting the risk of infection.

Use a similar trick to protect finger injuries. Just cut off all the rubber "fingers" except the one for your bandage. Now you still have finger traction, but your wound is protected.

DANDRUFF

Natural fixes nix the itch

You may blame the snowdrifts covering your shoulders on dry skin, but oil and an overgrowth of a common fungus are more likely culprits.

The yeast *Malassezia ovalis* thrives in oily areas, like your scalp, forehead, eyebrows, cheeks, and around your nose and ears. It lives on the skin of most people harmlessly, but in some, it grows out of control, causing your body to shed skin cells three times faster than normal. These dead, oily cells clump together, forming the scaly flakes known as dandruff or seborrhea.

Some people used to think if you took a dandruff flake out, painted it black, and placed it back on your head, all the white flakes would go away. Today, experts know managing flakes mostly means practicing good hair hygiene.

Wash daily. Since dandruff is linked to an oily scalp, washing your hair more often could be the only remedy you need. Try a gentle shampoo every day and see if flakes disappear.

Hold off on hairspray. Styling products like hairspray, gel, and mousse can build up in hair, even irritating your scalp if you have sensitive skin.

Try an OTC. Consider an over-the-counter medicated shampoo for tough-to-shake flakes. Some work by attacking scalp fungus, others by slowing the rate of cell turnover. Look for one containing selenium sulfide (Selsun Blue), zinc pyrithione (Head & Shoulders), coal tar (Neutrogena T/Gel), ketoconazole (Nizoral A-D), or salicylic acid (Ionil).

Be aware that cold weather, stress, illness, and being tired can all trigger a flare-up. Talk to your doctor if your dandruff doesn't clear up after several weeks of self-treatment. You could have a suppressed immune system, a more serious skin condition like psoriasis, or suffer from a neurological disorder like Parkinson's disease. She can diagnose you and prescribe stronger medicine to control stubborn flakes.

Sun sheds light on dandruff

A little sunlight on your head could help fight flakes, by curbing yeast growth. That's one reason you might have seen your dandruff improve in summer. Dermatologists say ultraviolet rays from the sun improve seborrhea in most people, though it can aggravate the condition in a few. Practice moderation, and wear sunscreen on your

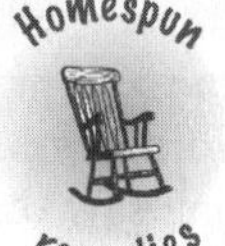

Household vinegar sweeps away flakes

Tap into vinegar's legendary healing power with this popular folk remedy.

- Combine 1 part apple cider vinegar with 1 part water.
- Spritz on your scalp with a spray bottle and gently massage in, being careful to avoid your eyes.
- Wrap a towel or shower cap over your hair and let the vinegar sit for 15 to 60 minutes.
- Rinse off and shampoo as usual.

Try this daily until dandruff disappears, then once a week to prevent flare-ups.

face and body. Skip the sunlight remedy if you use a dandruff shampoo made with coal tar, since this ingredient makes you more likely to burn.

'Tea' of a tree helps ditch dandruff

The healing power of a natural fungus-fighter could put an end to snow-topped shoulders. Scientific studies show using a shampoo containing 5 percent tea tree oil controls flakes as well as using a medicated shampoo made with ketoconazole (Nizoral) or an antifungal solution like Lamisil, containing terbinafine. Wash with it every day for the best snow control, and leave the shampoo on for at least three minutes before rinsing. Just watch out for any signs of an allergic reaction. And never use full strength tea tree oil, which can irritate your skin.

Aloe: shake the flakes and face the world

You can get rid of those annoying facial flakes with a safe, natural remedy – aloe vera. The same gel from this plant that soothes burns also gently improves the flaking and itching of facial dandruff, without harsh chemicals. In one study, people spread a cream made with 30 percent aloe extract on scaly spots twice a day for four to six weeks. Amazingly, more than half saw their seborrhea improve or disappear completely. To see what this natural anti-inflammatory and potent fungus-fighter can do for you, try smoothing aloe gel from the plant's leaf on flaky areas, or look for a topical aloe ointment in herbal shops.

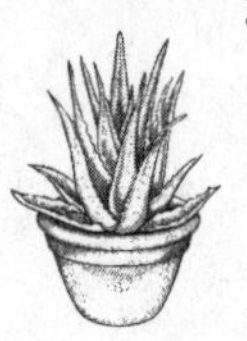

Aloe vera plant

Olive oil revives your tresses

Rub warm olive oil into your scalp to soften and loosen dense, scaly flakes before shampooing. Leave the oil on overnight to soften especially thick dandruff and comb out flakes in the morning. While you're at it, give your scalp a gentle massage to encourage blood circulation. Rub with your fingertips, not your nails, to avoid breaking the skin.

A salty scalp spells relief

A sprinkle of salt in your hair before shampooing can get rid of embarrassing dandruff. The natural abrasiveness of salt helps exfoliate your scalp and remove dead skin. Add a dash along hair roots and gently massage. Follow up with a shampoo and rinse.

Sweet treat dismisses dandruff

Want to dramatically improve your dandruff? Reach into the pantry for your honey jar, an excellent antifungal agent and possibly the only remedy you'll need. It worked for people with seborrheic dermatitis, an inflammatory skin disease that can include dandruff.

Every other day, they diluted raw honey with a bit of warm water then gently rubbed it on the affected areas of their face and scalp for two or three minutes. They left the honey on for three hours before rinsing off with warm water.

Within a week, the greasy scales were gone and itching had eased. After two weeks, the skin lesions were completely healed. Those who stopped the treatment saw their flakes return within a few months, but people who kept applying honey once a week were still flake-free six months later.

DEPRESSION

Cheer up with self-help remedies

Nothing seems fun anymore. You feel sad and tired most of the time. Sometimes you can't even manage to pull yourself out of bed in the morning. You have more than a slight case of the blues – you're experiencing depression.

Depression and other mood disorders affect about 20 percent of Americans at some point in their lives. Types of depression include major depression, the milder dysthymia or chronic, and atypical depression, in which people may not experience the usual symptoms. No one knows exactly what causes depression, but genetic factors, B vitamin deficiencies, traumatic events, and other illnesses may be to blame. Chemical imbalances in the brain – involving the neurotransmitters serotonin, dopamine, and norepinephrine – also play a key role.

It's important to recognize the signs of depression, both in yourself and in those close to you who may need help. Be on the lookout for these symptoms:

- feelings of sadness, grief, guilt, worthlessness, and helplessness
- loss of interest in activities you once enjoyed
- sleep problems, including insomnia or oversleeping
- decreased energy and fatigue
- changes in appetite and weight, whether it's significant loss or gain
- trouble concentrating, thinking, or making decisions

- restlessness
- thoughts of death and suicide

To overcome major depression, you probably need professional help. This usually involves cognitive behavioral therapy, antidepressants, or a combination of both treatments. But for cases of mild to moderate depression, there are effective, self-help remedies. Read on to discover how you can pull yourself out of the doldrums.

Popular beverage perks up your spirits

Coffee gets you going in the morning – and it may help keep you going. A 10-year study of 86,626 nurses found that women who drank two to three cups of coffee a day lowered their risk of suicide by 66 percent compared to women who never drank coffee. Four or more cups a day led to a 58-percent dip in suicide risk. So brew a pot of java – it's a cheap, easy way to perk up your mood. Because many

Mythbuster: Is depression all in your head?

Depression affects more than your mood – it also affects your body. A recent Canadian study found that people with depression were four times as likely to develop neck or back pain than people who weren't depressed. Pain and depression go hand-in-hand. People with painful conditions, like arthritis or fibromyalgia, often experience depression, too. Several conditions, including thyroid disease, stroke, obesity, and headache, have also been linked to depression. Studies show being depressed also means having a more difficult and shorter old age, whether because of heart attack, stroke, dementia, or osteoporosis.

people with depression have trouble sleeping, avoid drinking coffee – or other beverages containing caffeine – too close to bedtime.

Fish sends depression reeling

Floundering with the blues? Eat some flounder. Or serve up some salmon, tuna, mackerel, or herring. You could deep-six depression by adding fish to your diet. The essential fatty acids found in fatty, cold-water fish, called omega-3s, play a major role in brain function. Studies show they may even boost your mood.

A groundbreaking Harvard study found that fish oil helped people with bipolar disorder, or manic depression – a condition marked by extreme highs and lows. Other researchers have noticed low rates of depression in countries with high fish consumption, like Japan. A recent Finnish study found that women who rarely ate fish were more than twice as likely to be depressed than women who ate fish regularly. Fish oil may even help people who do not respond to standard antidepressants, according to a recent British study.

How does fish help? Experts remain unsure. The omega-3 fatty acids in fish may fight depression by reducing inflammation, boosting levels of serotonin, or keeping cell membranes fluid so neurotransmitters – your brain's messengers –can get through and deliver their messages.

If you're an absolute landlubber who can't stand fish, don't worry. You can also get omega-3 from walnuts, flaxseed, and dark green, leafy vegetables like spinach, arugula, kale, Swiss chard, and collard, mustard, or turnip greens.

Exercise keeps the blues on the run

It's hard to hit a moving target. So get moving, and make it harder for depression to hit you. Recent studies show that exercise can be just as effective as antidepressants or therapy in battling depression. It's also much cheaper.

Melt away tension

Progressive muscle relaxation calms your mind and your body. Here's how to do it. Find a quiet, comfortable place to sit. Take a few slow, deep breaths. Close your eyes and gradually relax the muscles of your body, one group at a time. Begin by clenching the muscles of your toes while you count to 10, then relax them for a count of 10. Enjoy how it feels to be relaxed. Move to tensing and relaxing your leg muscles, then on through the other muscle groups in your body, including your abdomen, chest, arms, shoulders, neck, and face. By the time you get to your head, you should feel much calmer.

In a Duke University study of 156 people age 50 or older, those who biked, jogged, or walked briskly for 30 minutes three times a week had similar success in overcoming depression as the other groups in the four-month study. One of the groups took the antidepressant Zoloft, while another group exercised and took Zoloft. The big difference came in the relapse rates. Only 8 percent of the people in the exercise group experienced symptoms of depression again, compared to 38 percent of those taking Zoloft and 31 percent in the combination group.

Further evidence for exercise comes from a University of Texas Southwestern Medical Center study. People who worked out for 30 minutes on a treadmill or stationary bike three to five times a week for 12 weeks reduced their symptoms of depression by nearly 50 percent. Researchers noted that results were similar to other common treatments, such as medication or cognitive behavioral therapy. The key is how many calories you burn in a week – not how often you exercise. But following the public health recommendations of at least 30 minutes of moderate exercise on most – and preferably all – days of the week should do the trick.

Beware of a dangerous combination

If you're taking a type of antidepressant called monoamine oxidase (MAO) inhibitors, you need to watch your diet. These drugs, which include phenelzine (Nardil) and tranylcypromine (Parnate), should not be taken with foods or beverages high in tyramine. Otherwise, you may experience a sudden, extreme spike in blood pressure known as a hypertensive crisis. Watch out for tyramine in aged cheeses, red wine, beer, very ripe bananas, sauerkraut, chicken livers, and aged or smoked meats. Tyramine can also be found in nasal decongestants and cold or allergy medications.

Music puts a song in your heart

Dust off your record player, pop in a compact disc, or turn on the radio, and you'll soon be singing a happier tune. Music therapy, which involves playing instruments, singing, or simply listening to music, can help you feel better. It not only eases depression, it reduces pain and stress and helps you sleep.

One study found that listening to music helped reduce depression by up to 25 percent in people suffering with chronic pain. Whether they listened to soothing selections chosen by music therapists or just their favorite songs, their depression improved. Music therapy might even help your antidepressants work better.

Supplements fend off the blahs

Prescription antidepressants improve your mood – but they may also come with unpleasant side effects, including nausea, dizziness, drowsiness, headaches, dry mouth, constipation, or diarrhea. Save money and sidestep side effects with these natural alternatives.

St. John's wort. Studies show this popular herbal supplement works as well as standard antidepressants – with fewer side effects – at a fraction of the cost. A one-month supply of St. John's wort costs around $10. The standard dose is 900 milligrams (mg) a day.. You can take two 450-mg doses or three 300-mg doses. Look for standardized formulations. Otherwise, you're not sure what you're getting.

St. John's wort

Remember, St. John's wort should only be used as a short-term treatment for mild to moderate depression. Major depression usually requires prescription drugs. Do not take St. John's wort if you're already taking a prescription antidepressant. A dangerous reaction called serotonin syndrome could result. St. John's wort may also interact with other drugs, so it's important to let your doctor know you are taking it.

S-adenosyl-methionine. Another promising supplement to keep an eye on is S-adenosyl-methionine, better known as SAM-e. Used for decades to treat depression in Europe, SAM-e was approved by the U.S. Food & Drug Administration in 1999. Your body naturally makes this compound and uses it to build the neurotransmitters serotonin, dopamine, and norepinephrine.

Some studies show SAM-e works faster, with fewer side effects, than prescription drugs. However, questions remain about the short length and the methods of many of these studies, some of which used injections instead of pills. Before trying SAM-e, you might want to wait for more conclusive research. Experts also warn not to use SAM-e to treat bipolar disorder, or manic depression.

Light therapy brightens your outlook

Winter brings more than snow, holidays, and colds. For people with seasonal affective disorder (SAD), the winter months and their lack of sunlight can bring on depression. Researchers think changes in the levels of certain brain chemicals, like serotonin, might be responsible.

Because darkness seems to trigger SAD, it makes sense that light therapy could help cure it. Although not much solid research exists, the few well-designed studies do support this theory. In fact, light therapy seems to help people with regular depression as well as those with SAD. Light therapy may even work as well as some antidepressants.

The key is the bright artificial light, measured in units called lux and delivered through a special light box. Typical therapy is at 10,000 lux and involves sessions lasting from 30 minutes to two hours a day. Just sitting near the light box does the trick. You could read, listen to music, or watch TV. Usually, early morning is the best time for light therapy.

You can buy 10,000-lux light boxes on the Internet or in some drugstores or hardware stores. Prices range from $200 to $500. Some health insurance companies will cover the cost.

Light therapy does come with some safety concerns. Possible side effects include headache, eyestrain, nausea, and agitation. Make sure you talk to your doctor before trying light therapy on your own.

Scents soothe troubled mind

Maybe you can't figure out how to snap out of your sad mood – but your nose knows. There's evidence your sense of smell can play a role in relieving certain forms of depression. That's the idea behind aromatherapy, a complementary medicine that uses the essential oils of plants. Scents commonly used to treat depression include lavender, basil, sandalwood, rose, jasmine, rosemary, patchouli, chamomile, bergamot, and geranium. When using essential oils, remember a little goes a long way. For a relaxing bath, combine 5 to 10 drops of essential oil with an ounce of carrier oil, like almond, apricot, jojoba, or grapeseed, and add it to your bath water.

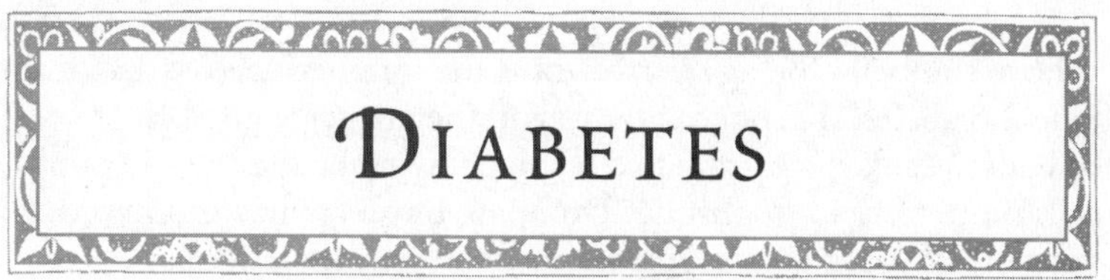

DIABETES

Real solutions for blood sugar problems

How about a powdered mouse for breakfast? Or a sulfur-molasses concoction at lunch? It's amazing what people once thought would cure diabetes. Luckily, experts now know what causes this disease and how to control it. Here's how it works.

Glucose, the most common type of sugar, is the fuel your body runs on, like gasoline in your car. Most of it comes from the foods you eat, including sugars and starches that break down into glucose in your digestive tract and get absorbed into your bloodstream. A rise in blood sugar triggers your pancreas to release insulin. This hormone grabs on to cells and moves sugar from your blood into each cell where it gets used as fuel. This system works great – unless something goes wrong.

- Type 1 diabetes. In this type of diabetes, your immune system attacks and destroys the pancreas cells that make insulin. This happens most often in childhood, although in rare cases it strikes adults. People with type 1 must take insulin several times a day.
- Type 2 diabetes. Once called adult-onset diabetes, type 2 develops gradually and mostly strikes adults. Your pancreas may no longer make enough insulin to move sugar into your cells, or your cells may become resistant to insulin and can't use it effectively. Either way, you end up with dangerously high levels of glucose in your blood.

High blood sugar can damage your nerves, eyes, kidneys, and blood vessels. If you have type 2 diabetes, you can dodge this fate by making a few key changes in how you live.

Lose the belly. Being overweight is the number one risk factor for type 2 diabetes. The more you weigh, the greater your risk. Scientists think the extra fat cells somehow make the rest of your cells more resistant to insulin. Dropping those pounds can improve your blood sugar control, blood pressure, and cholesterol.

Get moving. Exercise can help you lower your blood sugar, blood pressure, and triglycerides, as well as boost insulin sensitivity, slash your heart disease risk, and help you lose weight. In fact, exercising is just as effective as dieting at dropping pounds and improving blood sugar and insulin levels.

Try to get at least 30 minutes of physical activity most days, whether walking, gardening, or swimming. Aim for an hour if you're trying to lose weight. But talk to your doctor first. You may need to avoid certain types of exercise if you already have nerve and blood vessel damage in your feet and legs caused by diabetes.

Stop smoking. Men who smoked 20 or more cigarettes a day faced a 70-percent greater chance of getting diabetes than nonsmokers and former smokers in a study of more than 21,000 men.

More than 90 percent of people with diabetes have type 2. This chapter focuses on preventing and treating type 2 diabetes, though some of the same remedies may help type 1.

An aspirin a day keeps heart disease at bay

Cardiovascular disease, which includes heart attack and stroke, is the leading cause of death in the United States. On top of that, having diabetes can double, triple, even quadruple your risk. Fortunately, your medicine cabinet holds a simple solution.

The American Diabetes Association recommends men and women over age 40 who have diabetes take a daily, low-dose aspirin (75 to 162 milligrams) to cut their risk of heart attack and stroke. Unfortunately, most people who could benefit from aspirin therapy aren't using it. Often, they opt for treatment with fancier, more expensive statin drugs. But studies show aspirin reduces heart disease risk as well as statins at a fraction of the cost.

Experts think people with diabetes produce too much thromboxane, a chemical that narrows blood vessels and causes blood platelets to clump together. This can lead to blood clots and narrowed arteries. Aspirin keeps your body from using thromboxane and makes platelets slippery so they don't stick together.

Aspirin therapy is not right for everyone, especially people who bleed easily, have liver disease, or take blood-thinning medications. Talk with your doctor before trying it.

Tea: brew a cup of powerful antioxidants

Wouldn't it be nice if drinking a hot, soothing beverage every day could chase away diabetes? You're in luck, because evidence links both green and Red Bush teas with amazing protective powers.

Excess glucose in your blood reacts with oxygen to produce free radicals, unstable molecules that wreak havoc, particularly on your blood vessels. If you have diabetes, you have more free radicals floating around than other people, more than your body can get rid of on its own. These extra free radicals are the main culprits behind the serious complications people with diabetes face, such as heart disease, kidney damage, nerve damage, and diabetic cataracts and vision loss.

That's where antioxidant-rich foods, like green tea and Red Bush tea, come in. They give your body extra ammunition to disarm free radicals and, in the process, might protect you from developing diabetic complications. Here's the lowdown.

Red Bush tea. Red Bush, or rooibos, tea comes from the needle-shaped leaves of the *Aspalathus linearis* bush native to South Africa. True to its name, it makes a fragrant cup of reddish brown tea with more antioxidants than black tea, and it's caffeine free. Best of all, it might prevent vision loss caused by diabetic retinopathy and cataracts by keeping a lid on the amount of free radicals in your blood and eye lenses. Experts recommend drinking tea made from green, or nonfermented, rooibos leaves since they pack the most antioxidants.

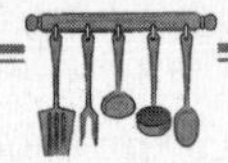

Steep green tea for 3 minutes in hot, but not boiling, water. Drink it before it cools and turns brown – a sign the antioxidants have stopped working. Steep rooibos tea for 5 to 10 minutes. Unlike green tea, the longer it steeps and the hotter the water, the more antioxidants you get.

Green tea. In a Japanese study, men and women who drank six or more cups of green tea a day were 33 percent less likely to get type 2 diabetes. Other teas, including black tea and Chinese oolong tea, didn't offer that protection.

The researchers think the caffeine in green tea may be partly responsible, but likely so are its rich stores of antioxidants known as catechins. In lab studies, green tea catechins protected diabetic red blood cells from oxidative damage. That's why experts think eating catechin-rich foods could help people with type 2 diabetes ward off long-term complications. Other research shows green tea improves how your body uses and stores glucose. These findings suggest it could prevent type 2 diabetes or lower your risk by controlling after-meal blood sugar spikes. Green tea might also help treat high blood sugar in people with existing diabetes.

A hearty breakfast beats disease

Mom was right – breakfast is the most important meal of your day. British researchers found starting the day off with a healthy breakfast before 8 a.m. lowered total as well as "bad" LDL cholesterol and improved postprandial, or after-meal, insulin sensitivity in women. Skipping breakfast, on the other hand, was linked to future weight gain.

What you eat also plays a big role. These breakfast foods can actually help fight diabetes, so start making them part of a healthier lifestyle.

Whole-grain cereal. Sitting down to a bowl of cereal can make you feel like a kid again. Eating cereal for breakfast seems to lower blood cholesterol and cut down the amount of fat and cholesterol you eat throughout the day. Whole-grain cereals, in particular, slash LDL and total cholesterol and boost insulin control, benefits refined grains don't boast.

Processing, or refining, makes the carbohydrates in grain easier to digest, so their sugar enters your bloodstream in a burst. This causes post-meal spikes in your blood sugar and insulin that, over time, can lead to type 2 diabetes.

Whole grains digest more slowly, and research shows their insoluble fiber improves your insulin sensitivity and could help stave off diabetes. Eating just three servings of whole grains a day can trim your type 2 risk 20 to 30 percent. It also slashes your risk of metabolic syndrome, a group of health problems that increase your risk of diabetes, heart attack, and stroke. So what are you waiting for?

Low-fat milk. The milk you pour on your cereal adds another layer of defense. In a 10-year study of nearly 40,000 middle-age and older women, eating low-fat dairy foods frequently reduced the risk of developing type 2 diabetes. Women who ate the most dairy were 21 percent less likely to get the disease than those who ate the least. Focusing on low-fat dairy products earned them even more protection – a 36-percent lower risk. Men fared similarly well in a separate study. Out of more than 41,000 middle-age and older men, those who ate the most dairy foods each day enjoyed a 23-percent lower risk of type 2 diabetes, with low-fat and skim milk packing the most protection.

Coffee. It may be the only addiction that's good for you. Study after study suggests a morning cup of joe keeps diabetes at bay, especially in people at high risk for the disease. Most recently, Japanese researchers followed 17,000 men and women for five years and discovered drinking three or more cups of caffeinated coffee each day scored them a 42-percent drop in type 2 risk, compared to drinking less than a cup a week. In this study, caffeine seemed to have its own protective powers, but coffee contains nutrients, like magnesium, and the antioxidant phenol chlorogenic acid that could help ward off diabetes.

Regular coffee temporarily dulls your insulin sensitivity if you don't normally drink it. This effect fades after a few days, but experts warn against taking up the habit in hopes of preventing diabetes. In fact, some studies suggest decaffeinated coffee drinkers get similar benefits.

Zesty spices balance blood sugar

Spices do more than season your food. They contain potent compounds that can treat disease. Scientists are currently studying these three spices for their power to battle diabetes.

Fenugreek. One of the oldest medicinal plants, fenugreek shows promise in lowering blood sugar levels for people with type 1 or type 2 diabetes. The seeds are rich in a soluble fiber that might help by interfering with the way your body absorbs sugar from food. And fenugreek is packed with an amino acid that stimulates your pancreas to release insulin. This exotic seasoning is found in curry powder, or you can buy the seeds separately. Some experts suggest eating 5 grams, about one and one-third teaspoons, of whole seeds daily. Watch your blood sugar closely if you take insulin or other diabetic medications, as adding fenugreek could cause hypoglycemia or low blood sugar.

Chili pepper. Adding a dash of cayenne pepper livens up food while dampening after-meal insulin spikes. Australian researchers seasoned the food of 36 people, who were overweight, with cayenne chili pepper. After four weeks of eating the spicy food, their insulin and blood sugar levels were measured. Daily doses of this spice evened out insulin levels and lowered blood sugar spikes after eating. People in this study added 16.5 grams, a little more than three tablespoons, of a cayenne chili spice blend to their meals each day.

Hidden danger of popular spice

Turmeric, the main ingredient in curry powder, can aggravate gallstones and bile duct blockages. Skip it if you have a history of gallbladder problems, or if you take blood-thinning drugs, like warfarin, since it can boost their strength.

Turmeric. Years of poor blood sugar control can lead to cataracts. But turmeric, the yellow spice in curry powder, can put the brakes on cataract growth. This pungent spice seems to protect your eyes from damage caused by high blood sugar. Use it to liven up rice, beans, and sauces. For the most benefits, add a dash of black pepper to your dish and drink a cup of green tea with your meal. You'll absorb up to 20 times more curcumin, the active ingredient in turmeric.

3 supplements take aim at diabetes

Three common supplements could turn the tide against diabetes with amazing results, from bringing down blood sugar levels to increasing your insulin sensitivity. Watch your blood sugar closely to avoid low blood sugar if you try any of these supplements.

Chromium picolinate. Normally, insulin attaches to muscle cells, prompting them to absorb and use sugar. In pre-diabetes and diabetes, these cells become resistant to insulin. Chromium picolinate supplements can help muscle cells become sensitive to insulin again and use sugar more efficiently.

This mineral may work especially well when taken with diabetes drugs known as sulfonylureas. In a recent study, people with diabetes taking 500 micrograms of chromium picolinate twice daily along with a sulfonylurea drug for six months showed great results. They became more sensitive to insulin, achieved lower blood sugar, and gained less weight than people with diabetes using sulfonylurea treatment alone. The study participants took Chromax brand chromium picolinate supplements made by Nutrition 21.

Ginseng. Feeling tired all the time? Try ginseng. This traditional Chinese medicine is found not only to lower blood sugar in people with type 2 diabetes, but also raise energy levels. Studies have found it may cut both fasting and after-meal blood sugar levels, plus lower your three-month average levels. What's more, ginseng appears to be a powerful antioxidant that could prevent diabetic vision loss and kidney complications by protecting delicate blood vessels from oxidative damage.

Most studies use American ginseng (*Panax quinquefolius*). Experts usually recommend taking 1 to 2 grams of raw ginseng daily, or 200 milligrams of ginseng extract made with 4 to 7 percent ginsenosides, the active ingredients. Try it for three weeks and monitor your blood sugar carefully to see if it works. Ginseng seems safe long-term, but women with a history of breast cancer should avoid it since it may stimulate breast cancer cells to grow.

MythBuster: Say goodbye to sweets?

Too often, people with diabetes feel sentenced to a lifetime of bland food. Not so, says the American Diabetes Association. You can still enjoy sweets and high-carbohydrate treats. The key is moderation.

Most people with diabetes can eat three to four servings of bread, potatoes, pasta, or other starchy foods daily, in small portions. In fact, whole-grain starches boast lots of fiber, which keeps your digestive tract healthy. Sweets are OK, too, if you eat them in moderation, exercise regularly, and eat an overall healthy diet.

Cinnamon. You don't have to suffer a heart attack just because you have diabetes. Cinnamon can help you control blood sugar, cut triglycerides, and lower total cholesterol, according to some studies. The theory – a compound in cinnamon called methylhydroxy chalcone polymer acts like insulin in your body. Insulin regulates your blood sugar, but it also helps control your cholesterol and triglyceride levels.

People who saw the best results in studies took cinnamon supplements rather than eating it in food. Dr. Richard A. Anderson, a researcher with the U.S. Department of Agriculture, says your saliva harms cinnamon, so eating it straight from the container likely won't help. In fact, taken this way the spice can build up in your body with potentially harmful results. Stick to supplements, and don't make the mistake of eating cinnamon oil. It's poisonous even in small amounts.

Smart steps pamper tender feet

If the shoe fits without rubbing, wear it. Blisters and cuts take longer to heal when you have diabetes, and they can easily turn into dangerous foot ulcers. Take good care of your tootsies.

- Wear thick, soft, cotton-acrylic blend socks to cushion your feet and pull moisture away from your skin. Avoid 100-percent cotton socks.
- Cut your toenails straight across and file down sharp edges.
- Wash your feet each day, but avoid soaking them in hot water.
- Sprinkle foot powder between your toes if you have sweaty feet to prevent fungus growth.
- Check daily for blisters, cuts, sores, or swelling. Use a hand mirror to look at the soles of your feet, or ask a friend or family member to help.

Diarrhea

Say 'stop' to a going problem

One minute you feel fine, the next you're racked with cramps, bloating, nausea, gas, and too many trips to the bathroom. How did things go so wrong so quickly? Blame it on whatever is forcing your bowels to work too fast, turning your colon into a rapid transit system. When waste speeds through your body, your intestine walls have less time to pull water from it, and the result – loose stools. Find the villain and you could get better. Consider this lineup of suspects.

Any number of intestinal diseases can cause chronic diarrhea – the kind that lasts longer than three days. It usually means you have a problem in your digestive system and you need a proper diagnosis from your doctor.

Short-term diarrhea, on the other hand, comes and – well – goes, lasting no more than three days. It may be a side effect of antibiotics or other medication. You might have food poisoning or traveler's diarrhea from sneaky little *E. coli* or other bacteria that contaminate food and water. Diarrhea can even come from food allergies, stress, bacterial and viral infections, or parasites. If you're suffering from this kind of no-frills diarrhea, you can help your body fight back with these steps.

- Bypass foods that are greasy, high-fiber, or high in fat. Don't drink alcohol or caffeine.

- Eat only soft, carbohydrate-rich foods at first. Start with the BRAT diet – bananas, rice, applesauce, and toast. Crackers and cooked cereals may also be safe.

- Drink plenty of fluids with electrolytes – potassium and sodium – so you don't get dehydrated. Good choices include clear sodas, fruit juice, broth, and, if you can tolerate it, chicken rice soup.

Here's an important word about over-the-counter anti-diarrhea medicines. Don't use them if you suspect a parasite or bacterial infection has caused your misery. Diarrhea is your body's way of purging these dangerous creatures. But, if you have severe diarrhea plus signs of dehydration, go ahead and use an anti-diarrhea product – but also call your doctor. Dehydration can be fatal.

When diarrhea turns dangerous

Most cases of diarrhea only last a day or so, but see a doctor if you have:

- diarrhea that lasts more than three days.
- severe stomach pain.
- blood in your stool or vomit.
- a fever of more than 101 degrees Fahrenheit.
- signs of dehydration, including dark urine, urinating less often than usual, fatigue, dry skin, lightheadedness, or confusion.

Probiotics: win the battle of the bugs

Any gardener worth his salt knows good bugs in the garden keep the bad bugs under control. Oddly enough, a similar trick can help prevent diarrhea. Several hundred species of bacteria live in your intestines. Some are "good bugs," called probiotics, which help maintain your health, and some are "bad bugs" that can cause infection and disease. If the balance between the number of good and bad bugs is thrown off, you can suffer from things like diarrhea. Fortunately

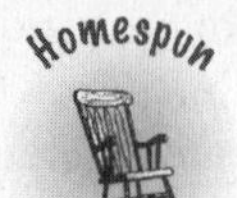

Swedish remedy 'berries' diarrhea

A folk cure from Europe's snowy Scandinavia may put the chill on diarrhea. Buy dried blueberries or make your own by spreading fresh ones in the sun until they wrinkle up. Store these little blue gems until your next diarrhea attack. Then measure out about 3 tablespoons and enjoy.

adding probiotics back into your body restores the balance and may help you feel better. You can get them from yogurt, probiotic drinks, or probiotic supplements. Here's how they might help.

- Antibiotics often cause diarrhea because they kill off good bugs and give bad bugs the upper hand. Ask your doctor how to use probiotics to resist antibiotic-caused diarrhea. Just avoid taking probiotic supplements within two hours of taking any antibiotic.
- If you get diarrhea from a virus that's "going around," probiotics might help you get well much sooner. Choose ones with names that begin with *Lactobacillus* or "*L.*" and start taking them as soon as your diarrhea begins. In general, try yogurt containing the probiotic *Lactobacillus casei* to prevent diarrhea.

Before you purchase probiotic supplements or dairy products, read the label. Stick to yogurts that promise "active cultures" or "live cultures" right on the package. Also, check supplement labels to see which probiotics they contain and how many you get. You need at least 1 billion probiotic bacteria a day.

Hidden laxatives can spell tummy trouble

Seemingly harmless foods could be the cause of your mysterious diarrhea, experts warn. Your trigger might be the natural fructose in grapes, honey, pears, or apple juice. Perhaps you're under sneak attack from a sweetener in candies, mints, and sugar-free foods – sorbitol, for instance, is notorious for its diarrhea-causing powers.

But that's not all. Notice whether you have trouble with the Olestra in fat-free potato chips or the lactose in milk, yogurt, and soft cheeses. And beware of other surprise offenders like table sugar or the caffeine in colas, coffee, and tea.

Try keeping a food and symptom diary every day. You may soon spot a hidden laxative lurking in your meals. Remove it from your diet and your diarrhea may leave along with it.

Eat greens without turning green

Children couldn't believe their luck in 2006. Spinach containing *E. coli* bacteria had made people so sick that all spinach was banned for days. Although safe spinach quickly became available again, you still need to know how to avoid food poisoning. These tips can help.

- To destroy *E. coli*, sauté or boil leafy greens at 160 degrees Fahrenheit or higher for at least 15 seconds.
- In the grocery store, choose fresh or bagged produce only if it is refrigerated or surrounded by ice.
- Place meat, poultry, and seafood in separate bags from fresh produce.
- If you buy produce that is already cut or peeled, refrigerate it when you get home.
- Know which varieties of whole fruits, veggies, and greens should be stored in the fridge. Ask your grocer.
- Wash fruits and veggies before peeling or eating. Dry with a clean paper towel.
- Notice which utensils, cutting boards, dishes, or counter tops you use when preparing meats,

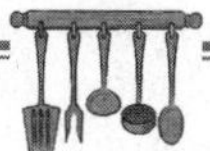

Make your own kitchen sanitizer by mixing 1 teaspoon of chlorine bleach into 1 quart of water. Spray your counter tops and cutting boards every so often to kill harmful bacteria.

fish, or poultry. Wash all of them with soap and hot water before using them for anything else.

Mighty mineral speeds recovery

Add more calcium to your diet if you're worried about traveler's diarrhea or food poisoning – researchers think it may protect you from this unpleasant condition. For 10 days, half the men in a Dutch study added an extra 1,100 milligrams of dairy calcium to their daily diet. Half did not. Then they were all infected with the *E. coli* bacterium. The extra calcium group recovered more quickly – probably because the calcium prevents *E. coli* from settling in and multiplying in your gut. You can easily get this amount. Drink a glass of skim milk, eat a Swiss-on-rye sandwich, sprinkle some grated mozzarella over a salad, and add fruit to one 8-ounce container of nonfat plain yogurt.

Psyllium calms a cranky colon

You may know psyllium best as the super constipation-fighter in Metamucil, but it can also relieve diarrhea. Because each tiny seed is coated with a natural gummy substance called mucilage, which absorbs incredible amounts of water, it makes your stool firmer. Studies show that psyllium can also encourage hasty intestines to move stool more slowly, giving your body time to reabsorb even greater amounts of water.

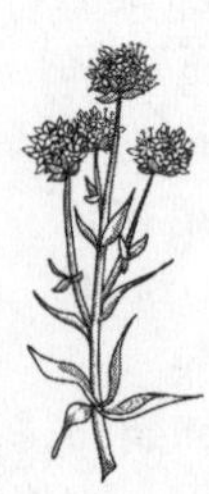

Psyllium

Talk to your pharmacist before you try psyllium. It may not be safe if you take blood-thinners like warfarin, medicines for diabetes, and many other prescription drugs. But if your pharmacist approves, try a product containing psyllium, like Metamucil, for three to seven days. For diarrhea, experts recommend taking anywhere from seven and one-half grams of psyllium up to 30 grams every day. Just remember to take each dose with plenty of water.

5 ways to thwart Montezuma's revenge

It can ruin a good trip while you're on it, or the memory of one once you get home. Traveling to high-risk areas – Mexico and Latin America, Africa, the Middle East, and Asia – can mean up to a 50 percent chance of developing traveler's diarrhea. It's caused by any number of microorganisms and will leave you with diarrhea, nausea, cramps, bloating, fever, and fatigue. But take these steps and you may prevent symptoms both during and after your travels.

- Before you go, ask your doctor what vaccinations and other medical preparations you need.
- Carry small packets of powdered rehydration solutions and a container of bottled water while traveling.
- Only eat thoroughly cooked meat, chicken, or shellfish, and only if they are served hot.
- While you travel, avoid the following local items: tap water, ice cubes, raw fruits and vegetables that cannot be peeled, food or drink from street vendors, and unpasteurized milk and dairy products.
- Drink only boiled or bottled water or carbonated drinks in sealed containers.

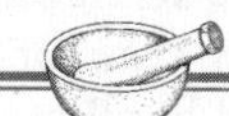

Think pink to help prevent traveler's diarrhea. Pink for bismuth subsalicylate of course – also known as Pepto-Bismol. Health experts say it can kill bacteria that cause food poisoning. Just chew two tablets after each meal and at bedtime while you travel.

Dry mouth

Super strategies can stimulate saliva

Used to be, nothing said dry mouth like being called on in Chemistry class, or coming face-to-face with the cutest boy in town. You could hardly swallow, let alone speak. Now that you're older, that dry-as-the-Sahara feeling could mean many things. But it's nothing to ignore. You need saliva, which is mostly water, to help digest food, protect your teeth, chew, and swallow. Saliva also keeps your mouth lubricated and guards against infection by washing away bacteria, viruses, and yeasts.

When you suffer from dry mouth, also called xerostomia, your salivary glands do not produce enough saliva. This makes it difficult to swallow, eat, or even talk. It also leaves your mouth wide-open to tooth decay and infections. Lack of saliva can affect your sense of taste and even cause a burning sensation or pain in your mouth. Without enough moisture, your lips or tongue can also become chapped or cracked.

This uncomfortable condition is most often a side effect of medication. In fact, more than 400 drugs – including antihistamines, blood pressure drugs, and antidepressants – can dry you out. But certain health conditions can also lead to dryness, like diabetes, hepatitis C, Parkinson's disease, and depression. If you've recently undergone radiation therapy, you may notice this side effect, as well. There's even an autoimmune disorder, called Sjogren's syndrome, in which your white blood cells attack your body's moisture-producing glands.

So, if dry mouth is more than just a passing nuisance, see your doctor. She may prescribe drugs like pilocarpine (Salagen) or cevimeline (Evoxac) to make your salivary glands work better. But there are many things you can do to feel less parched.

- Sip water throughout the day, especially with meals to help you swallow.
- Use a humidifier to moisten the air at night.
- Practice good oral hygiene. That means brushing your teeth at least twice a day with fluoride toothpaste, flossing, and seeing your dentist at least twice a year. While this advice applies to everyone, taking care of your teeth is especially important for people with dry mouth.

Chewable remedy wets your whistle

Battling dry mouth is as easy as walking and chewing gum at the same time. Actually, it's even easier because you don't even have to walk. Simply chew gum and you get your saliva flowing. Just make sure you choose sugarless gum. If you don't have a toothbrush handy, it also serves as a good substitute for brushing your teeth after a meal. Add extra moisture to your mouth by sucking on sugar-free hard candies, lemon drops, frozen grapes, Popsicles, ice chips, or a cherry pit.

Artificial saliva: short-term relief

Say you live in a country that does not produce oil. You can import what you need from an oil-rich nation. By the same token, if your salivary glands do not produce enough saliva, you can always import some. Artificial salivas – as aerosols or liquids – help moisten your mouth and make it easier to talk, chew, and swallow. But they don't contain the digestive and antibacterial enzymes found in real saliva. You'll also have to use them often, because they provide only temporary relief. You can find over-the-counter saliva substitutes, like Salivart, in most pharmacies.

Kitchen picks: what dries you out

A dry mouth can make you thirsty, but don't grab just any beverage. Some, like drinks with caffeine – coffee, tea, or soda – will only make you feel more parched. If you're after a snack, stay away from spicy or salty foods. These can be painful to your dry mouth and cracked lips. You're already at increased risk of tooth decay because you don't have enough saliva, so avoid sugary or sticky foods. That means cutting back on cookies and candy. Alcohol will dry you out as well, and it's often "hidden" in surprising places, like mouthwash. You'll want to read labels carefully. Try to remember all the naturally juicy foods you can enjoy and don't fret over ones that make a bad situation worse.

Easy-to-swallow tips improve mealtime

When you have dry mouth, eating can be a chore. The whole process of chewing and swallowing may seem like more trouble than it's worth. Instead of skipping meals – and skimping on nutrition – try these tactics from the American Dietetic Association.

- Drink your liquids through a straw.
- Eat soft, bland foods cold or at room temperature.
- Put your fruits and vegetables in a blender.
- Serve soft, cooked chicken or fish.
- Eat cereal with plenty of milk.
- Snack on slushies.
- Use broth, soup, sauce, gravy, butter, or margarine to moisten your food.

With these strategies, you can stop dreading dinner – or breakfast and lunch – and enjoy a meal that goes down easy.

Bark not worth the bite

Need a cure for dry mouth? Don't go barking up the wrong tree. The bark of the yohimbe tree, native to West Africa, contains a substance called yohimbine that may help – but may not be worth the risk. Studies show yohimbine can boost saliva levels in people taking tricyclic antidepressants, which tend to dry out your mouth. However, these studies used pure yohimbine, which you can't get without a prescription. You can buy a supplement called yohimbe bark extract, but it typically contains little yohimbine so it's unclear how helpful it would be. It also may interact with several medications and certain herbs and foods. To be safe, wait for more studies of yohimbe bark extract before giving this supplement a try.

Lip balm locks in moisture

You would love to kiss dry mouth goodbye – but your lips are too dry and cracked. Soothe those painful, parched smackers with a simple trick. First, moisten your lips with water. Then apply an oil-based lip balm or lipstick. That should lock in the moisture and keep your pucker smooth and kissable. Other options for keeping your lips moist and healthy include petroleum jelly, cocoa butter, ointments containing vitamin E, or a commercial product like ChapStick. Once you moisten your lips, try keeping them zipped. Breathing through your nose can help prevent your mouth from drying out.

DRY SKIN

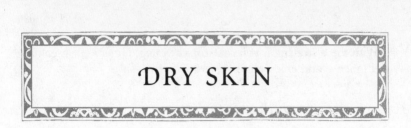

Put a damper on dry-skin blues

When you were a teenager you battled oily skin and pimples. Now the breakouts are long gone, but you're stuck with skin so dry you could use it as sandpaper. Why can't your body get it right?

Dry skin is one of the most common complaints of people as they age, mostly because your skin's sebaceous glands make less and less oil after puberty. However, your doctor may diagnose your trouble as a symptom of eczema or atopic dermatitis. Or it could be related to another health condition. For instance, if you suffer from asthma, hay fever, kidney disease, or diabetes, dry and sensitive skin can also be a problem. Women tend to have problems with dryness earlier than men because of hormone changes. For most people, the problem is worse in the winter when air is dry.

Besides being plain annoying, dry skin can bring on other problems, too. You may itch so bad you injure your skin with scratching and cause an infection. There's no magical cure, but you can follow some basic principles to keep skin comfortably hydrated.

Wonderful water: dryness relief inside and out

Think of your dry skin as being really, really thirsty. Here are three ways your body uses water to quench that thirst and replenish your skin's moisture.

Drink eight to 10 glasses of water daily. This simple fix adds moisture to your skin from the inside out.

Increase humidity in the air. Your dry skin problems may intensify in the winter because there's usually less moisture in cold air. To make things worse, indoor heating units dry out the air even more. When the air is dry, water is pulled out of your skin into the atmosphere. You can make your home or workplace more comfortable by using a vaporizer to add steam to the air, or a humidifier, which increases air moisture without using heat. Aim for a 50 percent relative humidity level. Many devices have a built-in humidity gauge.

Practice smart bathing. Some doctors say to bathe every other day so you don't wash away your skin's protective natural oils. No matter how often you bathe, keep these tips in mind.

- Use water that's warm instead of hot to avoid stripping oils from your skin.
- Keep a bath or shower short, about five to 10 minutes.
- Use a gentle skin cleanser instead of deodorant soap, which can dry skin.
- Pat yourself dry with a towel – don't rub too hard.
- Slather on moisturizer soon after bathing to lock water into your skin.

Cocoa: new secret to sensational skin?

A daily serving of dark chocolate may be just the ticket to battle dry skin. Flavanols, natural chemicals found in certain cocoa products like dark chocolate, work to increase blood flow to your skin, and battle thinning and dryness. A 12-week test showed women who drank a certain type of high-flavanol cocoa every day had skin that was less scaly and dry, and was less sensitive to damaging sunlight. To get these results, the women enjoyed the equivalent of about three and a half ounces of dark chocolate each day. This study was small, so your doctor is going to want more tests before writing a prescription for

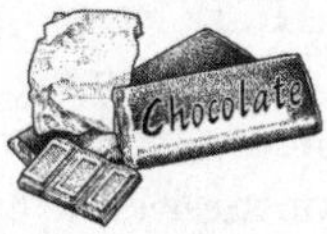

Epsom salt makes dry skin drier

Don't soak your tired, aching feet in an Epsom salt bath if your piggies are dry. This chemical compound – also known as magnesium sulfate – is an astringent, which means it will pull water out of your skin. You'll lose precious moisture where you need it most. Some experts say to try liquid soap with added skin softeners in your footbath, instead.

chocolate bars. But the results back up what experts already know – certain food compounds help your body from the inside out.

Moisturizers that make you say, 'ahhh!'

How do you know what lotion or cream to buy for your dry skin? Basically, decide what your most troublesome symptoms are and pick a moisturizer to fight that problem. Most contain a combination of three types of ingredients.

Softening agents change skin cells. Your outer layer of skin contains certain proteins called keratin. You can actually change these proteins with softening agents so they feel smoother. Look for urea, lactic acid, or allantoin on the label's ingredient list. Products with helpful softening agents include Jergens Ultra Healing Lotion or Neutrogena Norwegian Formula Foot Cream.

Humectants pull water into the skin. Ingredients like glycerin and propylene glycol are also known as hydrating or moistening agents. These work by pulling water out of the air or from your skin's lower layer to moisturize your epidermis, or outer layer of skin. Try St. Ives Mineral Therapy Body Moisturizer or Olay Quench Body Lotion.

Emollients keep moisture from escaping. Like a film of oil floating on a still pond, an emollient forms a barrier on your skin to keep that all-important moisture from evaporating. Look for lanolin, petrolatum, or mineral oil on the label of products like Vaseline Intensive Care Advanced Healing Lotion or Lubriderm Daily Moisture Lotion.

In fact, doctors say petrolatum – more often known as plain old petroleum jelly – is the best and cheapest moisturizer for dry skin. It doesn't cause allergies, and it's powerful enough to fight dryness on your lips – a tough place to keep moist. Petrolatum is a main ingredient in products for chapped lips like ChapStick and Carmex. No matter what moisturizer you choose, slather on plenty and use it often.

3 tips to topple the itch

Unbearable itching, or pruritus, may be the most annoying thing about dry skin. To keep it at bay, doctors say to avoid using laundry detergent with too many additives and dryer sheets. Both can leave itch-inducing chemicals in your clothes. And check your diet. Lots of caffeine, alcohol, or spicy foods expand tiny blood vessels to bring out your skin's sensitive side. Above all, if you have an itch, don't scratch. You can damage your skin, make the itch even worse, and bring on infection. Try these tricks instead.

- Wrap with a cool compress. A bit of a chill is more likely to soothe your itchiness than a hot bath, which can make the irritation worse.

- Rub on an ice cube. Besides bringing cooling relief to the area, an ice cube has little chance of scratching and damaging your skin.

- Take the vinegar cure. Cover your dry, itchy area with a cloth soaked in vinegar. Leave it on for about 20 minutes to kill bacteria and help moisturize your skin. Or add anywhere from two tablespoons to two cups of vinegar to your bath for the same effect.

Earaches

Tricks to tame painful ears

You might be surprised at what can cause earaches. Even when your ears are healthy, problems with your sinuses, tonsils, teeth, jaw, or throat can give you an earful of pain. But earaches are just as likely to be a sign of infection. To ease the pain, take aspirin or acetaminophen, and ask your doctor to pinpoint the problem. After all, the more you know, the better you'll be able to help yourself.

Two leading causes of earaches are middle ear infections and outer ear infections. Middle ear infections are a plumbing problem. Your middle ear sits behind your eardrum. Normally, a "drainage pipe" called the Eustachian tube keeps your middle ear free of fluids. This tube is also the ventilation shaft that prevents air pressure from building up against your eardrum.

But colds, allergies, or flu can cause swelling that blocks your Eustachian tube. This traps fluid in your middle ear and encourages infection-causing bacteria to thrive. It also causes symptoms like earache, dizziness, ringing and stuffiness in the ears, hearing loss, fever, and headache. If the infection is severe, your eardrum may rupture, causing the trapped fluid to leak from your ear. Call your doctor if this happens.

Outer ear infections work differently. These infections are sometimes called swimmer's ear because water in your ears invites bacteria to grow. Those bacteria can also start an infection if something breaks the skin in your ear canal. A simple scrape while cleaning your ear can be enough to wreak havoc. You'll know when an infection starts because you'll have symptoms like earache or itchy ear, thick ear drainage, stuffiness in your ear, swelling, dulled hearing, ringing in the ear, and even more pain when you touch or pull on your ear.

If you get frequent ear infections, see your doctor. Otherwise, use these tips to keep your ears healthy.

- Wash your hands often with soap and water to avoid colds and flu.
- After swimming or bathing, tilt your head and pull your earlobe in different directions to let water out. Then gently dry them with the corner of a tissue or use a hair dryer on low power held at least 12 inches away from your ear.
- Don't clean your ears with a cotton swab or any item that could scrape your skin. These may push earwax deeper into your ear or open the way for bacteria.
- Get treatment for severe allergies.

Symptoms that need your attention

Ear infections usually aren't serious. But, if you've taken aspirin or acetaminophen and still have a fever of 102 degrees Fahrenheit, get medical help. You also should see your doctor if you have any of these symptoms.

- a severe headache or discharge from your ear
- worsening of dizziness or hearing loss
- weakness on one side of your face
- ear pain lasting several days
- swelling or increasing pain around your ear
- continued symptoms after antibiotic treatment

- Limit or avoid using earplugs for swimming or bathing unless your doctor approves. They trap water in your ears.
- Don't smoke.

Pillows fight nighttime pain

If lying down triggers earaches or makes them worse, grab a few pillows. Propping your head up seems to help your ears drain and might make you feel better.

Chewing gum: unwrap infection protection

Try chewing your way out of an ear infection. Researchers discovered that kids who chewed gum sweetened with xylitol were less likely to get ear infections. Xylitol, a natural sweetener found in certain fruits, hinders the growth of bacteria notorious for causing ear infections. Some health experts think chewing gum sweetened with xylitol might also help grown-ups.

Several studies suggest getting at least 6 grams of xylitol daily, spread out over the day. Four sticks of a high-xylitol gum, like Carefree Koolerz, every day should do the trick. Gums with sorbitol and other sweeteners probably don't contain enough xylitol to help prevent ear infections. If you can't find high-xylitol gum, ask your dentist where to find it. Xylitol might also help prevent cavities.

Household combo silences swimmer's ear

Two items nearly everyone keeps around the house – rubbing alcohol and white vinegar – could help keep you from getting swimmer's ear, even if your only "watering hole" is the bathtub.

Make your own eardrops using equal parts of white vinegar and rubbing alcohol. The rubbing alcohol helps dry your ear, while the white vinegar makes your ear canal more acidic. Not surprisingly, ear-infecting fungus and bacteria won't stick around.

MythBuster: Are eardrops safe?

Although eardrops are often used to treat ear infections and other ear problems, they can cause damage if you have a ruptured eardrum. Don't take chances. Check with your doctor before using eardrops.

After swimming or bathing, put a few drops in each ear and wiggle your ear lobe. Wait a few moments and then tilt your head to let the drops drain out. But don't use these drops if you already have swimmer's ear or a tear in your eardrum, and stop using them if they cause stinging or pain.

Valsalva maneuver unsticks 'glue ear'

Your ears can get stuffy and clogged even if you don't have an ear infection. It happens when fluid gets trapped behind one or both eardrums. In severe cases, the fluid is very sticky, which causes a condition called glue ear.

Fortunately, an easy trick called the Valsalva maneuver can bring speedy, temporary relief from that "underwater" feeling. Before you try it, make sure you don't have an ear infection. To start, take a deep breath. Hold your breath while you close your mouth and pinch your nose shut. Then blow your nose very gently for a few seconds. Your ears should open right up.

Top tips for travel trouble

Vacations should be fun, but driving in the mountains or flying in planes can make your ears hurt – thanks to air pressure. Even in a pressurized airplane cabin, your ears are affected by air pressure changes as you take off and land. If your Eustachian tubes are blocked because of a cold or allergy, they can't keep the pressure inside each ear equal to the pressure outside, so your ears hurt.

For relief, try chewing gum or eating candy. Both make you swallow, which stimulates a muscle that helps open your Eustachian tubes. If you don't have candy or gum, try yawning, swallowing, or the Valsalva maneuver. You can also consider buying filtered earplugs specially designed to help keep equal pressure on both sides of your eardrum.

If you have a cold or allergies, ask your doctor what to do before you go on a trip. If she says it's OK for you to fly, ask her to recommend a decongestant or antihistamine to help keep your Eustachian tubes open.

Ear candles: don't get burned

At first, ear candles don't sound so bad. Their sellers claim lighting one end of this long, hollow candle pulls air up from the unlit end – much like a campfire sends smoke upward. The sellers also say this creates suction, which draws wax out of your ear canal. But there's a catch.

To use an ear candle, you lie on one side, stick the candle in your ear, and ask someone to light the other end. Unfortunately, this has caused burns, ear injuries, and blockages of melted candle wax in people's ears. Even worse, tests have found no evidence these candles help remove earwax or ease ear infections.

Gentle warmth stops earaches cold

Your house may be full of drug-free earache relievers. You can use a washcloth soaked in warm water, a hot water bottle wrapped in a towel, or a first-aid gel pack warmed in hot water. Or try a heating pad set on its lowest setting. But think like Goldilocks when preparing your favorite ear warmer. Make sure it isn't too hot before you press it to your ear and always re-warm it as soon as it starts cooling off.

FATIGUE

Easy steps lead to more energy

Sometimes it's simple to understand why you're tired. Working long hours, exercising too hard, or not getting enough sleep can leave you exhausted. But what if you feel tired all the time, for no obvious reason? That's the mystery people with chronic fatigue syndrome (CFS) face every day.

Besides a constant lack of energy, CFS – which affects about four in every 1,000 people in the United States – comes with the following symptoms.

- short-term memory loss
- inability to concentrate
- sore throat
- muscle pain
- headaches
- swollen lymph nodes
- sleep that doesn't refresh
- painful joints

Often, CFS starts with a simple cold or the flu. However, instead of clearing up after a few days, the symptoms linger for months or even years. While some researchers believe an infection triggers this condition, no one knows for sure what causes it. Genetic and psychological factors, brain or immune system abnormalities, and exposure to chemicals may all play a role.

Get a diagnosis. Because chronic fatigue syndrome shares so many symptoms with other diseases, it's difficult to diagnose. Doctors will first rule out other conditions, including infections like mononucleosis and the Epstein-Barr virus, or autoimmune diseases like lupus and multiple sclerosis. Depression can cause similar symptoms – but depression and CFS often go hand-in-hand. Other conditions that may occur with chronic fatigue include fibromyalgia and irritable bowel syndrome. Once you know you have chronic fatigue syndrome, what can you do about it?

Plan your course of action. Conventional treatment could include a combination of behavioral therapy and medication, such as antidepressants or over-the-counter pain relievers. But there are small decisions you can make every day to keep you feeling lively.

- Learn how to pace yourself and schedule your day accordingly.
- Make the most of the energy you have. For instance, don't waste energy standing when you can sit.
- Don't try to do too much. Set priorities, and keep expectations reasonable.
- Get things done when you feel most energized, and schedule naps when your energy is at its lowest.

Ask for help. Consider joining a support group for chronic fatigue syndrome. It may help to talk to other people who can understand what you're going through. While you're there, you can share these helpful tips for dealing with fatigue.

Food can refuel your engine

When the fuel gauge on your car's dashboard approaches "E," you know it's time to find a gas station. Similarly, your body needs fuel to keep running. Food satisfies your hunger and gives your body needed energy. But don't settle for junk food. A healthy diet is a key part of any treatment plan for chronic fatigue. For maximum energy, make sure you follow these eating tips.

Count on carbohydrates. With the recent popularity of the Atkins Diet, "carb" has become a four-letter word. But carbohydrates remain your body's preferred source of energy. In fact,

Homespun remedies

Scent-sational ways to wake up

Even when you're exhausted, you can muster enough energy to sniff. Make it the right fragrance and a whiff is all you need for an instant pick-me-up. The scent of lemon can stave off fatigue and keep you invigorated. Lavender, whether in a spritz or footbath, can revitalize you. Put the two together and aromatherapists say you've got one heady energizer. For when you're behind the wheel, try peppermint or cinnamon. These aromas are said to make drivers more alert and less frustrated.

restricting carbohydrates can leave you feeling worse and more fatigued after exercise. Complex carbohydrates, like those in whole grains and starchy vegetables, are best, but simple carbohydrates, such as those in fruits and honey, can give you a short-term energy boost. Aim to get both kinds into your diet.

Fish for healthy fats. Too much fat can be dangerous to your health, but the right kinds, in moderation, pack a healthy, high-energy punch. Replace saturated fat with polyunsaturated fat – found in safflower and sunflower oil – or monounsaturated fat – in olive oil, canola oil, and avocados. Omega-3 fatty acids, the kind found in seafood, may be especially helpful.

Pick good protein. Protein helps regulate how your body uses other sources of energy, like carbohydrates and fats. You can find protein in meat, fish, poultry, eggs, beans, nuts, and low-fat dairy products. But, again, moderation is key. According to the Institute of Medicine, only 10 to 35 percent of your total calories should come from protein. That means beware of high-protein diets. They may increase your risk of kidney stones, osteoporosis, heart disease, or stroke.

Fill up on fiber. A recent study found that eating high-fiber breakfast cereals, like Kellogg's All-Bran and Bran Flakes, reduced fatigue by 10 percent. Other good sources of fiber include whole grains, fruits, and vegetables.

Mind your minerals. Iron makes up hemoglobin and myoglobin, two compounds that carry oxygen throughout your blood and muscles. Without enough of this important mineral, you're bound to feel weak and listless. Good sources include meat, eggs, legumes, and dried fruit. Zinc not only boosts your immune system, but it produces energy from other nutrients. Try to get 8 to 11 milligrams a day from red meat, oysters, chicken, pork, fortified cereals, and beans. While it's better to get your nutrients from foods, consider a multivitamin/mineral supplement to fulfill your nutrition – and energy – needs.

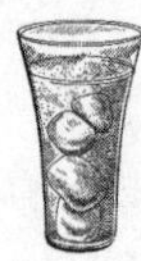

Drink up. Whatever you eat, make sure to wash it down with plenty of fluids, since dehydration is a major cause of fatigue. But don't feel you have to spend money on fancy sports drinks. These may help athletes, but for most people, plain old water works just fine.

In addition to what you eat, pay attention to when and how you eat. Never skip breakfast, which helps keep you alert and focused. Also, consider eating several small meals and snacks throughout the day, rather than three big meals. Your body uses lots of energy to digest large amounts of food sitting in your stomach. And concentrating all your resources on digesting can leave the rest of you feeling sluggish. Smaller portions, on the other hand, give your body a steady supply of fuel – so your personal energy gauge never reaches "E."

Caffeine: the pick-me-up that can let you down

You feel a little sluggish, so you reach for a big, steaming mug of coffee. Will the caffeine give you that burst of energy you need – or will it be more trouble than it's worth? The answer may be a little bit of both.

Caffeinated beverages, like coffee, tea, or soda, give you a temporary energy boost. For a short time, you may be more alert and productive, but caffeine's stimulating effect wears off in about two hours. What follows is a slump, similar to the letdown after a sugar rush. Besides feeling lethargic, you may also get a headache. Caffeine can lead to fatigue in other ways, too. As a diuretic, caffeine makes you go to the bathroom more often. This loss of fluids can put you at risk for dehydration, a major cause of fatigue. Caffeine can also keep you awake at night, so you don't get the restful sleep your body needs.

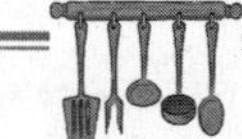

Try this energizing beverage as an alternative to coffee in the morning. Mix 2 cups each of grape juice, white grape juice, and apple juice. Add 1 cup of apple cider vinegar. Keep the mixture in the refrigerator, and pour yourself a glass to start each day.

Your best approach is to use caffeine wisely. Limit yourself to one or two caffeinated beverages each day – and make sure to drink them before 3 p.m. Keep in mind that caffeine is also found in chocolate and some over-the-counter pain medications.

Exercise revs your motor

Too much activity can be tiring – but so can doing nothing. If you don't move much during the day, your body's metabolism slows to a crawl, leaving you sluggish and fatigued. Luckily, you can overcome this with a smart approach to exercise.

You don't need to run a marathon or spend hours in the gym. Just 10 minutes of moderate exercise a day can boost your energy, reduce fatigue, and improve your mood. Try walking, jogging, swimming, cycling, or dancing, although any activity helps. Even a walk around the room or a quick stretch can get your blood flowing.

Several studies show that people with chronic fatigue syndrome can benefit from an exercise program. The key is to gradually increase your activity without overdoing it. Start slowly, with maybe 3 to 5 minutes of exercise, and find activities that suit your energy

MythBuster: Can supplements stop fatigue?

Many herbs and supplements wow you with advertisements promising to boost energy levels. Unfortunately, none of them have strong evidence to support their claims. On top of that, because the Food and Drug Administration does not regulate herbs or supplements, you can never be exactly sure what you're buying. The bottom line is you might buy a supplement that doesn't really work in the first place, or you could buy one that might work but doesn't contain enough of the right ingredients to do you any good. For the time being, be wary of supplements claiming to boost your energy, including St. John's wort, melatonin, comfrey, coenzyme Q10, and DHEA.

level. Every two weeks, add a bit more time and exertion, if you can. You may have an occasional setback, but don't give up.

Stress-busting strategies provide pep

When you feel stressed out, you also feel worn out. Stress – whether it comes from your job, family, or a medical condition like chronic fatigue syndrome – saps your energy. Here's one easy and healthy way to cope with stress and boost your energy – in 20 seconds. This gentle stretching exercise stimulates your nervous system and can be done anywhere, any time.

- Sit forward in a chair with your feet flat on the ground. While breathing out, stretch your arms straight in front of you until your palms touch, keeping them about shoulder-height. Roll your shoulders forward slightly and hunch your back.
- Still keeping your arms straight, open them wide to the sides, breathing in deeply. See how far behind you your arms can go without straining. Push your stomach and chest out, arching your back slightly.

- Bring your arms together in front of you again, breathing out. Slightly roll your shoulders forward and hunch your back. Rest and relax.

You can also try other deep breathing exercises, muscle relaxation techniques, stretches, biofeedback, or massage therapy. For stress relief that's no work at all, listen to music, watch a funny movie, keep a journal, or talk to friends or relatives.

Smart sleep habits keep you refreshed

You may think you can get by on less than six hours of sleep – but you may be doing more harm than you realize. Regularly skimping on sleep, night after night, can leave you feeling fatigued. Even if you don't feel sleepy, you build up a "sleep debt" that affects your ability to function. Give your body the rest it needs with these helpful tips.

- Stick to a sleep schedule. Go to bed and wake up at the same time each day.
- Keep your bedroom cool, dark, and quiet.
- Avoid foods that may cause heartburn and interrupt your sleep.
- Limit alcohol. A drink or two before bed may knock you out, but your sleep may be restless and unsatisfying.
- Do not smoke. Nicotine can keep you awake.
- Exercise early – not too close to bedtime.
- Relax before bed. Spend some time unwinding with soft music or a quiet activity.

If you don't get enough sleep at night, you can always nap during the day. A 15- to 20-minute nap can recharge your battery and give you the energy you need to complete the day. Just nap before 3 p.m. so you don't disrupt your evening sleep schedule.

FOOT ODOR

Secrets to sweet-smelling feet

Foot odor is all about sweat and bacteria. Your feet and hands have more sweat glands – about 3,000 per square inch – than any other part of your body. While this moisture evaporates from your hands, shoes and socks seal off your feet, making a warm, dark, moist place for naturally occurring bacteria to thrive.

Neither the bacteria nor the sweat smells bad alone. The unpleasant odor arises when the bacteria eat and digest the sweat. The secret to keeping feet sweet is to cut back both the number of bacteria and the amount of sweat on your feet and in your shoes.

- Use good foot hygiene. Wash them every day with antibacterial soap and lukewarm water. Dry them carefully, especially between the toes.
- Wear shoes made from materials that breathe, like natural leather or canvas. Avoid rubber and plastic.
- Change shoes and socks daily to keep them clean and dry. Always wear socks with closed shoes. Thick cotton socks are best to draw moisture away from your feet.
- Dust your feet regularly with foot or baby powder.

It's easier to fight foot odor when your feet don't sweat so much, but a genetic condition makes some people – especially men – sweat more than others. Stress, some medicines, hormonal changes, and the amount of water you drink also affect your sweat output. Talk to your doctor if you can't cure this condition yourself.

Simple steps stop stinky shoes

Often it's your shoes and not your feet that smell bad. Perspiration and bacteria generate just as much odor in your shoes as they do on your feet, so make sure your footwear is well ventilated. Wear open-toed shoes and sandals when you can, and stay away from tight shoes and boots.

You need to air out your shoes for at least 24 hours after each wearing, so don't use the same pair two days in a row. Alternate athletic shoes so they can dry between workouts. Always wear socks – especially when you exercise – to soak up moisture. If shoe odor won't go away, get rid of the shoes.

You can use baking soda, cornstarch, and essential oils to make an inexpensive, odor-absorbing foot powder. Sprinkle it in your shoes at night, shake them around to spread the powder, and dump it out in the morning. Or make reusable sachets from a handful of powder and the feet of an old pair of pantyhose. Fill, then tie off the ends and put them in your shoes each night. Replace the powder when it loses its pleasant aroma.

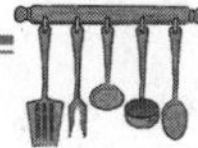

Make your own foot powder by stirring together 1/3 cup cornstarch or unscented talcum powder and 1/3 cup baking soda. Mix 15 drops cypress essential oil with 15 drops lavender essential oil and add this a drop at a time to the powder. Sift through a fine mesh strainer to blend the oils thoroughly. Add 10 to 15 drops orange or lemon oil for more fragrance.

Foot soaks wash away odor

A good soak not only makes your feet feel better, it can make them smell better, too. Just warm water and a little dishwashing solution will clean away sweat, bacteria, and dead skin cells that contribute to foul foot odor. Give your tootsies an even better aroma with additional ingredients.

- Epsom salt, sometimes called the ultimate foot soak, is actually magnesium sulfate. These mineral crystals absorb odors and smooth rough spots.
- Baking soda is famous for absorbing all kinds of odors, but it also neutralizes acids on your skin and helps wash away oil and perspiration.
- Add a few drops of essential oils that also act as natural deodorants – like cypress or tea tree. Some oils even have antibacterial or antifungal properties. Just never apply essential oils directly to your skin.
- For more potent antibacterial qualities, take advantage of the acetic acid in vinegar. Soak your feet for about 15 minutes in a solution of one part vinegar and four parts warm water.
- Black tea contains tannic acid, which kills bacteria and closes pores so your feet stay drier longer. Boil two tea bags in a pint of water for 15 minutes and then add two quarts of cool water. Soak for 30 minutes. Try this out every day for a week.

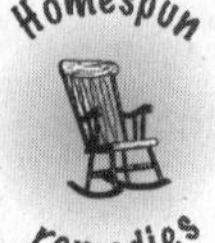

Top tips may freshen your feet

Feeling desperate? See if any of these folk foot-odor remedies work for you.

- Stick smelly shoes in the freezer or outside on a cold night to get rid of the odor.
- Put these things in your shoes overnight – a fabric softener sheet to deodorize or a tissue soaked in rubbing alcohol to kill bacteria.
- Use spray or roll-on antiperspirant on the bottom of your feet.

FOOT PROBLEMS

Home treatments soothe aches and pains

It's not surprising if you have sore feet. Each foot has 26 bones, 33 joints, and more than 120 muscles, ligaments, and nerves. As you get older, your feet widen and flatten, and the fat padding on the soles of your feet wears down. One study found that nearly nine out of every 10 seniors have foot problems.

When you walk, your feet support your weight, absorb shock, and keep you balanced. Every day, most people spend about four hours on their feet and take 8,000 to 10,000 steps. Women – probably because of high heels – are at greater risk than men for severe foot pain, which is a major cause of disability in older women.

Foot pain can come from ill-fitting shoes, natural changes in your foot's size and shape, high-impact exercise, poor posture, or any number of medical and hereditary conditions. Here are some common problems that can make your feet hurt.

Plantar fasciitis. When your heel hurts, it's likely plantar fasciitis. Tiny tears and inflammation in the tendons and ligaments, or fascia, that stretch from your heel to the ball of your foot cause the pain. It's a common problem, and it often happens to only one foot. Overuse during sports and exercise, poor-fitting shoes, or an uneven stride that puts too much pressure on your foot are possible causes.

Heel spurs. Calcium deposits under your heel bone, called heel spurs, can develop along with plantar fasciitis and add to the inflammation and irritation in your heel.

Little-known cause of Achilles pain

Sometimes pain and swelling in your Achilles tendon can signal a build-up of cholesterol. This common, inherited disorder, called heterozygous familial hypercholesterolemia (HeFH), prevents the removal of cholesterol from your bloodstream. Instead, it accumulates in your arteries – which leads to early heart disease – and in certain tendons. Scientists have found that many people complain of Achilles tendon pain long before HeFH is discovered. If your Achilles tendon hurts for no reason, ask your doctor to check your cholesterol.

Achilles tendonitis. Small tears can cause your Achilles tendon, which connects your calf muscle to your heel bone, to become inflamed, causing pain just above your heel. Overuse or strain injuries are likely culprits.

Bunions. These bony growths develop at the base of your big toe causing joint pain and redness. Tight-fitting shoes with pointed toes or high heels that put too much pressure on the front of your foot can cause bunions. Arthritis and heredity are also to blame.

Hammertoes. This permanent deformity of your toe joint causes your toe to bend upward slightly and then curl downward, resting on its tip. Eventually, the tendons contract and your toe stiffens into a hammer-like shape. Hammertoes occur most often to the middle toes when they don't have enough room to lie flat in your shoe.

You can do a lot to ease aches and pain at home with items you have in your pantry, medicine cabinet, or even your sock drawer. Always see a podiatrist, a foot specialist, for serious foot problems, and never treat your own feet if you have diabetes, heart problems, or poor circulation.

People with diabetes have special problems with blood vessels and damaged nerves, and they are more likely to be hospitalized for foot problems than any other complication. If you have diabetes, see a podiatrist at least once a year.

'Proper fit' the key to happy feet

Be kind to your feet when buying shoes. No matter how good they look or how stylish they are, don't buy them if you have to force your feet into them. You're asking for trouble from bunions, hammertoes, corns, heel pain, and a host of other problems if you don't wear shoes shaped the same as your foot.

New shoes should be comfortable right out of the box. If they fit well, they won't need to be "broken in." You should have a half-inch of space between your longest toe and the end of your shoe. The joint where your foot attaches to your toes should fit in the widest part of your shoe without being squeezed.

The next time you're in the market for a new pair of shoes, remember these essential tips:

- Shop at the end of the day when your feet are larger. You'll be less likely to buy shoes that are too tight.

Footprint test for flat feet

Flat feet can cause severe foot, knee, and leg pain. To find out if you have flat feet, step on a paper towel when you get out of the shower and look at your footprint. The area between your toes and your heel should be about half the width of the front of your foot. If that strip is wider, your arches aren't normal. See your doctor if flat feet are causing you pain.

- Measure both feet every time you buy shoes. Not only does your foot size increase as you get older, one foot is usually larger than the other. Fit shoes to your largest foot. The heel and the area across your instep should be snug, but not too tight.
- Try on both shoes and walk around on a hard surface. They should be comfortable, fit well, and have room for you to freely wiggle all of your toes.
- Look for shoes with wide toe room, sturdy heels, and cushioned insoles if you choose to wear high heels.

Stretch away heel pain

Plantar fasciitis is the most common cause of heel pain. In fact, it's responsible for a million doctor visits each year. Stretching, which restores strength and flexibility, is the best way to calm the pain and relieve stiffness. Try the following stretch three times a day, beginning first thing in the morning before you get out of bed.

- Sit on the side of your bed and cross the foot you want to work on over your other knee.
- Grasp your foot with the hand from the same side, fingers on the ball of your foot, and pull your toes back toward your shin until you feel a stretch in your arch.
- Hold for a count of 10 and repeat 10 times.

Regular, low-impact exercise, like walking, swimming, or cycling, can help, too.

Massage gives weary feet new life

A good foot rub might not fix your foot problems, but it will make your feet dance with joy. Massage relieves the soreness and discomfort from bunions, hammertoes, and worn-out feet. When muscles are fatigued, the chemical lactic acid builds up, irritating nerve endings. Massage steps up blood flow and gets rid of the lactic acid.

Herbal therapy for achy feet

Make your own foot massage oil from a few drops of cypress, lavender, or eucalyptus essential oil and a tablespoon of arnica oil, which is good for soothing aches and pains. Never use arnica on broken skin.

Try this simple massage. Using your thumb, index finger, and middle finger, rotate each toe. Then gently twist each foot like you were wringing a washcloth, moving the top and bottom in opposite directions.

Old standbys cool off pain

Two standard treatments – ice and nonsteroidal anti-inflammatory drugs (NSAIDs), like aspirin and ibuprofen – are still the best way to ease the pain and swelling of Achilles tendonitis and plantar fasciitis. Both of these remedies decrease blood flow to reduce the inflammation responsible for your distress.

You can make an ice pack by wrapping a towel around a plastic bag filled with ice and a small amount of water. Put it on the sore area for about 20 minutes at a time, two or three times a day. A damp towel left in your freezer for about half an hour makes a good cold compress. Use it to soothe sore bunions and hammertoes.

Insoles cushion every step you take

Learn a lesson from men and women who spend a lot of time on their feet. A study of New York police officers reported that six out of 10 had less foot pain when wearing insoles. Insoles, or shoe inserts, support your feet and act like shock absorbers when you walk or run.

You can buy many kinds of insoles – usually for less than $20 – at athletic stores and drugstores. They are particularly helpful to relieve plantar fasciitis and other heel pain. Some shoes have built-in insoles, so you may get relief simply by changing to another shoe brand.

For more serious problems, like fallen arches or abnormal foot structure, you may need a podiatrist to prescribe a pair of orthotics. These are custom insoles designed to fit your feet and relieve your specific problem, but they can cost $300 or more.

Experts suggest people with milder foot problems try the less-expensive, over-the-counter insoles before going to prescription orthotics. One study found 72 percent of people had less foot pain from store-bought insoles and only 68 percent from custom made.

MythBuster: Do magnets stop foot pain?

You'll have less pain from plantar fasciitis if you put magnetic insoles in your shoes, but it won't be because of the magnets. Researchers at the Mayo Clinic found that regular insoles work just as well as those with magnets. Every year Americans spend half a billion dollars on magnetic products because they believe magnets relieve pain by increasing blood flow or changing the way nerves signal pain.

GALLSTONES

Cast away stones for good

During the Middle Ages, people in Europe and Asia believed they could dissolve gallstones with a tea made from mugwort, the herb St. John wore as a belt. A few centuries later, lounging in the springs of Carlsbad was the way to ease the pain and pass the stone. Other "treatments" have included turpentine and opium. Fortunately, you have far better choices available today because experts have figured out how gallstones develop.

These stones are crystals that form from the liquid bile in your gallbladder. Your liver makes bile to digest the fats from foods, but your gallbladder stores it until the fats arrive in your intestines. Then, your gallbladder automatically squeezes bile through tiny ducts leading to the intestine, and fat digestion begins.

Bile naturally contains the raw ingredients for stones. In fact, gallstones get their start when too much cholesterol, bile salts, or bilirubin accumulate in the bile and are left to stagnate in your gallbladder. Then stones can form slowly and painlessly. They may be smaller than a grain of salt or grow to the size of a hen's egg.

Around 90 percent of gallstones never cause symptoms, but any stone that drifts into your ducts and causes a blockage can trigger inflammation, infection, and pain.

These gallstone attacks often happen after a delicious, high-fat meal. After all, fats cause your gallbladder to send bile into your ducts. So any gallstones lurking in that bile may lead to pain in the upper part of your midsection, which may even stretch out to your shoulder blades. You could also have bloating, gas, indigestion, and nausea.

You're more likely to get gallstones if you're over 50, overweight, or have high cholesterol. And women are more prone to them at any age. If you suspect you may be at high risk for stones or you've already had them, take these steps to help prevent them in the future.

- Eat fish instead of meat twice a week. The omega-3 fatty acids in fish lower your odds of gallstones, whereas meat raises them. Enjoying it twice a week limits your exposure to mercury and other toxins, as does choosing fish like salmon, herring, or sardines.
- Eliminate or cut back on saturated fat sources like butter, whole milk, cheese, fried foods, stick margarine, meats, and many packaged foods. Too much saturated fat raises cholesterol, the main ingredient in most gallstones. This fat also slows your digestion so gallstones have more time to form and grow.
- Replace some of your saturated fats with stone-stoppers like olive oil and flaxseed.
- Avoid foods that contain trans fatty acids, which may raise men's odds of gallstones.
- If you're overweight, seek out tasty food and fun exercise that helps you lose pounds. Weight around your middle raises your gallstone risk the most, but it's also the easiest to lose. Just don't try to lose more than one or two pounds a week. Rapid weight loss, crash diets, or repeatedly losing and regaining weight makes your liver produce extra cholesterol.

Surprising defense against stones

Rejoice if you're a coffee drinker. One study found coffee relieved symptoms in women who already had gallstones. Another discovered that men who drank two to three cups a day were less likely to develop the stones at all. And, according to the respected

Nurses' Health Study, women can slash their risk by drinking four cups of joe daily.

But don't reach for the decaf. Only caffeinated coffee seems to work, possibly because it stimulates gallbladder muscles and lowers the cholesterol in bile. On the other hand, caffeinated soft drinks seem to raise gallstone risk. So what should you do?

If you've never been a coffee drinker, experts recommend against guzzling java just to avoid stones. One study suggests it may not work, and coffee can be a poor health choice for many people. But if you already enjoy coffee daily, it may be an additional way to prevent gallstones or lessen their symptoms.

Fiber delivers triple protection

Imagine yourself at a farmhouse restaurant. The menu features sun-drenched fruits, field-grown vegetables, and hearty whole grains and beans. High-fiber foods like these pack a trio of gallstone defenders you don't want to miss.

First, you could order a whole grain like sweet corn or old-fashioned oatmeal. The insoluble fiber in these foods help your liver produce

Bag a double defense from tea

Not only do gallstones form in your gallbladder, they sometimes develop in the bile ducts that lead to your intestines. If these wandering stones cause a blockage, doctors may recommend gallbladder removal surgery. Fortunately, new research suggests that women who drink at least one cup of tea daily, especially green tea, lower their risk of both bile stones and gallbladder cancer.

less cholesterol-laden bile. That fiber also coaxes digestive products along, so gallstones have less time to form.

Second, you could order a bean and rice dish, peas, hummus, seeds, whole-wheat pasta, or whole-grain bread. The vegetarian proteins in these foods drive off gallstones, too.

Along with that, try a side of asparagus, or top off your meal with a sweet orange. Their soluble fiber latches on to bile and sweeps it out of your body. Many fruits, veggies, beans, and grains contain both soluble and insoluble fiber, so eat more of these regularly.

Nuts crack down on risk

You might not think of a peanut butter and jelly sandwich as gallstone-fighting nutrition, but guess again. Researchers say peanut butter, peanuts, and other nuts could slash your risk of gallstone-related surgery by 25 percent. Perhaps this works because nuts are low in saturated fats, but high in cholesterol-fighting "good fats" and fiber. Nuts also contain phytosterols, which may keep you from absorbing as much cholesterol from the foods you eat.

So start nibbling peanuts, walnuts, and almonds instead of gallstone-promoting saturated fats. Eat them in place of potato chips and other packaged snacks, or use them to replace some of the meat in casseroles, soups, and stews.

And, of course, treat yourself to a yummy peanut butter and jelly sandwich regularly.

Watch out for tasty trouble

Cinnamon rolls, yeast rolls, and other carbohydrates play a surprising role in forming gallstones. High blood sugar triggers your body to make more insulin, which raises the cholesterol that forms stones. A high-carbohydrate diet does the same thing. In fact,

Stones make 4 herbs hazardous

Talk to your doctor before trying dandelion, artichoke leaf, turmeric, or ginger. If you have gallstones, these herbs may not be safe.

research shows that people who eat more carbs have a higher danger of gallstones.

Avoid eating too many breads, cereals, potatoes, and other starchy foods, and keep sweets to a minimum. Items high in table sugar, fruit sugar, or starches may be particularly risky.

Experts also warn against high-carb, low-fat diets. These diets are a double whammy because a fat intake of less than 10 grams per meal could keep your gallbladder from emptying regularly, while high carbs help fill it with cholesterol. Cholesterol that's all dressed up with no place to go is more likely to turn into stones.

Critical vitamin crushes cholesterol

A sweet pepper a day could keep gallstones away. That's because a deficiency in vitamin C is linked to extra risk of gallstones. But you only need one sweet green pepper to get your minimum daily amount of vitamin C. Eat a red one, and you'll get twice the amount of vitamin C a woman needs each day.

This critical vitamin helps break down cholesterol so it can't turn into stones. Maybe that's why a study has shown that women with the highest vitamin C amounts in their blood have less risk of gallbladder disease. Get more vitamin C by eating foods like brussels sprouts, citrus fruits and juices, broccoli, kiwi, papaya, strawberries, and frozen peaches. And ask your doctor whether vitamin C supplements are right for you.

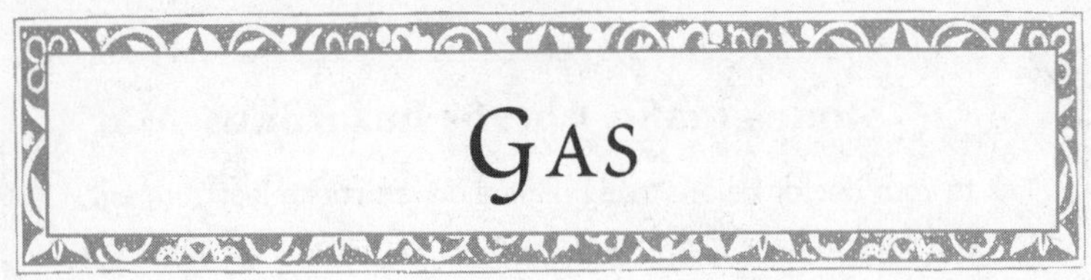

GAS

Deflate intestinal distress

You try to treat your body like a temple, but sometimes it feels more like a prison – complete with its own gas chamber. All that trapped air gurgling around in your gut makes you feel uncomfortable and bloated. Relief, when it comes, often has its own embarrassing sound effects. In some cases, gassiness can be a symptom of a more serious condition, such as gastroesophageal reflux disease (GERD), an ulcer, irritable bowel syndrome, or Crohn's disease. But more often than not, belching and flatulence do not signal anything more than a social blunder. In fact, passing gas anywhere from 14 to 23 times a day is considered quite normal.

Get the facts on gas. Gas sneaks into your body in two ways. First, you swallow air when you eat or drink too quickly, smoke, chew gum, wear loose dentures, or even sigh deeply. And then, some carbohydrates – starches, sugars, and soluble fiber – aren't completely processed until they reach your large intestine, or colon. There, bacteria finish breaking them down, producing gas in the process. Most of the gases, including hydrogen, carbon dioxide, and methane, are odorless. But the bacteria may also release sulfur, which has an unpleasant smell.

Stop gas in its tracks. Folklore has it, if you were born during a thunderstorm, you will suffer gas problems all your life. But don't despair. There's no reason you must endure one more day of this problem – no matter when you were born. There are, in fact, many helpful things you can do to avoid gas altogether.

☛ Eat slowly and chew your food thoroughly.

- Do not chew gum or suck on hard candies.
- Avoid carbonated beverages.
- Keep a food diary to pinpoint problem foods.
- Check with your dentist to make sure your dentures fit properly.
- Quit smoking.
- Sit up straight after eating.
- Try over-the-counter remedies, like Beano or products like Gas-X or Mylanta Gas containing simethicone, which combines small gas bubbles into larger, more easily passed ones.

There's no need to feel trapped by bloating, belching, or flatulence. Escape the gas chamber with the following tips.

Problem foods trigger gas attacks

Like John Dillinger or Pretty Boy Floyd, beans rank as the No. 1 outlaw when it comes to gas – and deservedly so. But they certainly

Dairy can be scary

That bowl of ice cream tastes great, but the gas that follows is no picnic. If dairy products bring on gas, bloating, and abdominal pain, you may be lactose intolerant. That means your body doesn't produce enough lactase, the enzyme responsible for digesting the main sugar in milk, called lactose. This uncomfortable condition, which affects up to 50 million Americans, is more common in blacks, Asians, and seniors. To deal with it, cut back on dairy until you determine how much you can tolerate. Some experts recommend eating yogurt with live active cultures to help you digest lactose. You can also buy lactose-reduced milk products or lactase supplements like Lactaid or Lactrase.

aren't the only potential troublemakers. Any food that contains soluble fiber, starches, or sugars – such as raffinose, sucrose, sorbitol, mannitol, and fructose – can give you gas. Besides beans, here are some other foods worth keeping an eye on.

- alcohol
- apples
- apple juice
- artichokes
- asparagus
- avocado
- bananas
- bran cereals
- broccoli
- brussels sprouts
- cabbage
- cauliflower
- corn
- cucumbers
- garlic
- grapes
- green peppers
- leeks
- lentils
- melon
- noodles
- nuts
- oats
- onions
- peaches
- pears
- potatoes
- prunes
- radishes
- raisins
- soybeans
- turnips
- watermelon
- wheat

Remember, not all foods affect everyone the same way. Something that may be a problem for you may pose no trouble at all for your spouse's digestive system. In addition, many of the listed foods are healthy so you don't want to avoid them entirely. Instead, pay attention to which foods affect you and cut back on those.

Go slow on fiber. While high-fiber foods – like fruits, vegetables, and whole grains – can cause a gas problem, fiber is extremely important for gastrointestinal health. The key is to add fiber to your diet gradually so your system gets used to it. Too much, too fast can lead to bloating and gas. Make sure to drink plenty of water to help fiber do its job. Aim for at least six glasses a day.

Trim the fat. Fatty foods can lead to abdominal pain and bloating even if they don't cause gas, themselves. That's because fat delays stomach emptying, which allows gas to build up. Cut back on these unhealthy foods to avoid the problem.

Get cooking. Many people find cooked vegetables easier to digest than raw. The cooking process breaks down some of the carbohydrates, giving the bacteria in your gut a head start.

You may not be able to completely sidestep gassy food "outlaws." But by identifying and limiting your problem foods and making a few simple changes, you can minimize the damage they cause.

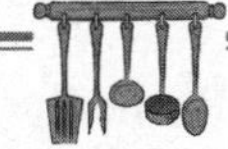

Get all the nourishing benefits of beans without the gassy side effects. First, soak your dried beans for about 4 or 5 hours, then drain. Cover with fresh water and boil for 10 minutes. Reduce heat and simmer for 30 minutes. Drain and cover with more water. Then simmer until beans are tender, about 1 to 2 hours. You can also try adding a few drops of Beano, an anti-gas food enzyme, to your cooked beans.

Exercise eliminates extra gas

Sometimes gas behaves like an unwanted guest who just won't leave your party. Only rather than bad jokes or boring conversation, your gassy guest dishes out bloating and pain. Luckily, you can speed gas along just by being more active.

A Spanish study confirms it – physical activity helps excess gas zip through your system. The researchers suspect exercise increases pressure on the abdomen, forcing gas out. Walking, jogging, cycling, and other activities can all nudge gas through your digestive tract. Try to exercise at least 30 minutes every day. Strengthening your abdominal muscles will also help prevent bloating. Pull in your stomach several times a day or do sit-ups regularly.

Fennel fights flatulence

Just as some foods promote gas, others counteract it. Take fennel, for instance. This herb has been used as a carminative, or anti-gas agent, for centuries. Its power comes from the oils found in the plant's seeds. In fact, Indian restaurants often place a dish of fennel seeds near the door to help with digestion. You can also get the benefits of fennel in tea form. Pour 8 ounces of boiling water over a half-teaspoon of crushed seeds and let it steep for 15 minutes. Or look for fennel teabags in stores. In addition to fennel, you can try these other traditional – and effective – home remedies.

Peppermint. Let this refreshing herb, which contains menthol, stimulate your digestion and relieve any intestinal spasms. Steep one tablespoon of leaves in hot water for a soothing tea that relieves gas and indigestion. Check with your doctor before using peppermint if you have liver or gallbladder disease.

Caraway. The seeds of the caraway plant add flavor to foods like cabbage while reducing their gassy side effects. A recent German study found an herbal preparation containing caraway, licorice, lemon balm, and peppermint completely soothed indigestion symptoms in almost half the people tested.

Homespun remedies

Home remedies take the pressure off

Researchers are not working furiously in laboratories to discover a cure for gas. So there's no sense waiting for the latest medical breakthrough. Instead, try soothing your system with traditional folk remedies such as a handful of anise seeds, a piece of ginger candy, or a cup of chamomile tea after dinner. You can also find relief in your spice rack or herb garden. Germans take cinnamon to treat indigestion, bloating, and flatulence, while traditional Chinese and Indian medicines rely on turmeric. The herbs made famous by Simon and Garfunkel – parsley, sage, rosemary, and thyme – have all been used to soothe indigestion or prevent gas.

Gout

Princely advice to battle the disease of kings

Living high on the hog can leave you aching in the joints from gout, especially for middle-age men and older women. This painful disease is caused when too much uric acid in your blood triggers crystals to build up in your joints. The result? Sudden pain, especially in joints of the toes and fingers.

Uric acid is normally made in the liver from purines, or nitrogen-containing compounds in some foods. Your body can make too much uric acid if you eat certain foods. People once thought gout only troubled kings and other wealthy folk who splurged on rich food and alcohol. That's why it's sometimes called the "disease of kings." Experts now know gout is a form of arthritis that tends to run in families.

Several kinds of drugs, like steroids and nonsteroidal anti-inflammatory drugs (NSAIDs), which include aspirin and ibuprofen, can help keep gout symptoms at bay. But there's a lot you can do to keep yourself symptom-free.

- **Watch your weight.** Losing some extra pounds if you're overweight and making wise food choices can make a big difference.
- **Keep your fluids up, heat down.** It's important to keep from getting dehydrated, since this can increase uric acid concentration in your blood. Avoid hot, humid weather and stay out of saunas.
- **Pack on the ice.** A simple but helpful treatment for a painful gout flare-up is keeping an ice pack on the affected joint. Try this for 30 minutes, four times a day to banish pain, swelling, and fluid build-up.

Dodge a serious gout complication

The same unhealthy diet that can lead to gout also puts you at risk for a heart attack. Researchers have shown a strong connection between the two problems. A study of about 13,000 men found that, after smoking and family history of heart disease, gout is the strongest risk factor for a heart attack. Uric acid encourages inflammation, which can result in blood clots that cause heart attack and stroke.

Although folk remedies for this ancient disease abound, you probably don't want to cook a poultice made from an anthill, and putting on your right sock first every morning may not do the trick. Read on to discover healing hints that gout sufferers like Isaac Newton and Benjamin Franklin would have loved to try.

Tiny fruit fights inflammation and pain

Who needs an excuse to eat cherries? If you do, think about their anti-inflammatory power. Tart and sweet cherries contain anthocyanins, antioxidants that reduce inflammation. Researchers tested this theory by having a group of women eat 45 fresh Bing cherries every day for breakfast. They found that levels of uric acid in the women's blood went down during the five hours after their fruity meal. Anthocyanins are especially useful in easing the severe pain of gout, but they can also help with other kinds of arthritis pain, so you may not need tons of pain relievers. If fresh cherries aren't in season, try dried cherries or cherry juice. Raspberries and blueberries also have plenty of anthocyanins.

Traditional gout diet still a great choice

Those who suffer from gout have heard the old advice to banish foods with lots of purines. Changing your diet may seem difficult, but following this time-tested recommendation is probably the best way to avoid painful flare-ups. Avoiding all purines in food would be nearly impossible, but here are some troublemakers you should stay away from.

- red meats, including beef, pork, and lamb
- soup, broth, and gravy made from meat
- organ meats, like liver
- canned tuna, shrimp, lobster, scallops, and anchovies
- chocolate
- alcohol, especially beer and liquor

Drinking wine in moderation seems to have no effect on uric acid levels. What's more, vegetables with lots of purines, like spinach, mushrooms, and pinto beans, don't seem to cause problems for people with gout.

3 ways to curb gouty symptoms

Sidestepping a gout flare-up isn't only about avoiding certain foods. Here are three simple, inexpensive ways to keep your symptoms under control.

Drink more water. Most uric acid leaves your body through your kidneys, so you want to keep them working well. Drinking plenty of water can help dissolve uric acid crystals, allowing them to be flushed out of your body.

Homespun remedies

Bathe away pain with vinegar

Vinegar is an old-time treatment for the pain and swelling of gout. Some people swear by soaking their painful feet in a bath of apple cider vinegar and warm water.

Pour yourself a cup of coffee. Research shows drinking coffee can lower the uric acid level in your blood to prevent gout's onset. One study found that men who drank coffee every day – even five cups or more a day – had the best results. Another study that included both men and women found similar results. Nobody knows why coffee has this effect, but other drinks containing caffeine, like green tea, don't reduce uric acid levels.

Enjoy low-fat dairy products. Your mother said milk would build strong bones, and it turns out good ol' dairy also helps your joints. For people with gout, getting more low-fat dairy products can help lower uric acid in the blood. Health experts aren't sure why, but they think milk proteins help break down uric acid. Also, it may be that eating and drinking lots of dairy products means you're eating less red meat and other purine-rich foods, which can trigger a gout flare-up. In one long-term study, men who drank two or more glasses of skim milk each day had the best results. Low-fat yogurt is also a great choice.

Vitamin C helps rout gout

Gout, a form of arthritis, can take hold when too much uric acid builds up in your blood, forming crystals in your joints that cause pain and swelling. Called the "king of antioxidants," vitamin C not only helps fight cancer and heart disease, researchers say it lowers uric acid levels.

Researchers tested the theory that large doses of vitamin C could remove the extra uric acid. Many years ago, they found that people who took 8 grams of vitamin C a day had lower uric acid levels after a week. But that's a lot of vitamin C – about 89 times the suggested daily intake for men. Recently, scientists checked to see if a lower dose of vitamin C might work. Sure enough, they found 500 milligrams a day reduced uric acid levels. Since you would have to eat more than seven oranges to get this much vitamin C, many health experts recommend taking a supplement.

GUM DISEASE

Easy ways to save your smile

You'll probably keep more of your teeth longer than your grandparents did. Advances in dental care, fluoridated water and toothpaste, and better diets mean today, only 20 percent of people between 55 and 64 years old have lost all their natural teeth. The bad news is gum disease is still a problem for about 90 percent of people at some point.

It all starts when mouth bacteria build up into a film on your teeth and gums. This is called plaque, and too much of it can creep below your gum line to make your gums swollen, red, and painful. Now you have gingivitis, or gum disease. If it gets bad enough, it's called periodontitis, and it can damage your bone and even cause you to lose teeth. Even worse, doctors see links between gum disease and other serious health problems like heart disease, diabetes, pneumonia, and stroke.

Now that you know gum disease affects more than just your mouth, you'll want to make changes to your whole way of life to avoid it. Good hygiene and good nutrition are key, but here are two other lifestyle decisions important to healthy gums.

Kick the habit. Smoking a pipe was an old folk remedy for a toothache, but it's the last thing you should do to care for your teeth and gums. Smoking causes at least half the cases of gum disease in the U.S. Any tobacco use, including chewing tobacco, can lower your immune system and make infection more likely.

Avoid alcohol. Perhaps a shot of whiskey used to be a common folk treatment for mouth pain, but drink to excess and you're more likely to develop gum disease.

A dentist or gum specialist – periodontist – can perform surgery and other treatments to combat advanced gum disease. But who wants to undergo an operation or lose their teeth? With good habits, you can prevent gum disease in the first place or keep early gum disease from turning into something worse.

Good hygiene keeps gums in the pink

Steer clear of advertising hype when it comes to gum care. Many fancy new – and expensive – tools and toothpastes are out there, often promising to clean better, make your teeth whiter, and even help you look younger. But you don't need gizmos and potions to keep your mouth healthy. You do need to follow the suggestions of the American Dental Association (ADA) concerning oral health.

Brush twice. Use fluoride toothpaste with the ADA seal of acceptance, and buy a good toothbrush. Although not all the bells and whistles are necessary, a power brush that rotates and oscillates reduced gingivitis by 17 percent in one study. Similarly, don't bother

Power brushing is a no-no

You don't need elbow grease to clean your teeth and gums. Researchers in Europe found brushing harder and longer doesn't remove more plaque. In fact, too much pressure with your toothbrush can damage your gums and even wear down your teeth. The study showed brushing for two minutes with medium force and a power toothbrush got rid of the most plaque. Do that twice a day for the best results.

with an expensive toothbrush sterilizer unless you have a lowered immune system. Instead, follow these rules.

- Don't share your toothbrush. Bacteria in your mouth cause tooth decay and gum disease, so keep yours to yourself.
- Rinse and tap your toothbrush after you use it to remove water and debris. Store it upright to air-dry – not covered or sealed.
- Replace your toothbrush every three or four months – sooner if the bristles look worn.

Floss every day. You know you should floss, so stop making excuses. Dentists say it is the best way to remove plaque from the crevices between your teeth. You may have seen some advertising claims that using mouthwash is as good as flossing, but don't believe them. Swishing with a mouthwash containing essential oils, like Listerine Antiseptic, can help fight plaque, but experts say it's no substitute for flossing.

See your dentist twice a year. Early gum disease often shows no sign, so let your dentist check. A special exam, called Periodontal Screening and Recording (PSR), can identify problems and keep tabs on your gum health. Your dentist will use a probe to measure how deep your gum pockets are. Deeper pockets give bacteria a place to hide and grow.

Guard your gums with a balanced diet

Most periodontists urge people to eat a well-balanced diet because it is so critical for healthy gums. But do you know just which nutrients are most important?

Try a trio of vitamins. These three, vitamins C, D, and folate, are especially helpful for avoiding gum disease.

- Early sailors sucked on limes so their teeth wouldn't fall out. They were after vitamin C, which helps rebuild collagen in bones and cartilage, and especially connective tissue in your gums. A large study found people who don't get enough vitamin C are more likely to have gum disease. Try getting your daily dose from citrus fruits, bell peppers, sweet potatoes, or cantaloupe.

- Vitamin D makes your teeth and bones strong, but now research suggests it helps battle gum disease in yet another way. Scientists think the anti-inflammatory powers of vitamin D control gum bleeding and swelling. Your body makes it from sunlight, but eat egg yolks, liver, or fortified milk for even more.
- You need folate to make red blood cells. It also seems to make your gums more resistant to irritation. If you don't get enough, you're at greater risk of developing gingivitis. You'll find plenty of this B vitamin in bananas, orange juice, avocados, and green leafy vegetables.

Consume lots of calcium. Don't get enough of this important mineral every day and you could double your risk of gum disease – probably because calcium strengthens the bone supporting your teeth. Most milk is also fortified with vitamin D, so this drink can do double duty.

Say sayonara to sugar. You could say the path to gum disease is paved with sugar. When sugars and starches in food build up on your teeth and gums, plaque-causing bacteria use them to grow. More plaque means more chances for gum irritation and gingivitis.

Grab some whole grains. Skip the white bread and potatoes and choose brown rice, dark breads, and other whole grains. A recent study found men who ate the most whole grains had less gingivitis. Some experts believe whole grains help control blood sugar levels, which influence oral health.

Enjoy antioxidants. Polyphenols, natural chemicals in some plant foods, work as antioxidants to reduce damaging waste from your body's cells – waste that may have a hand in destroying bone and tissue. Delicious sources of polyphenols include strawberries, blueberries, cranberries, red grapes, grape juice, tea, and red wine.

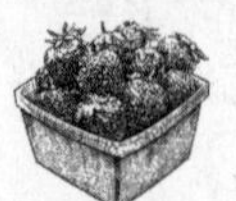

MythBuster: Raisins no good for gums?

Think the sticky sweetness of raisins means they're as bad as a candy bar for your teeth and gums? Not so. Oleanolic acid, a natural chemical in "nature's candy," stops the growth of two main types of bacteria that damage teeth and gums. It also keeps bacteria from sticking to surfaces in your mouth and building up as plaque. Researchers say this substance and two similar ingredients make raisins a better snack choice than processed goodies. Raisins also got a good score for oral health because they are sweetened by fructose and glucose – not cavity-causing sucrose.

Sugar substitute: sweet protection

It looks like sugar. It tastes like sugar. But it certainly doesn't act like sugar. In fact, experts insist it prevents cavities. Xylitol – say it like "xylophone" – is a natural sugar alcohol found in raspberries, strawberries, and plums. As an FDA-approved food additive, it sweetens chewing gum, candy, and toothpaste.

In more than 300 studies, researchers found it battles tooth decay and gum disease differently from antibiotics, which kill bacteria. Xylitol, instead, prevents bacteria from growing and attaching to your teeth and gums. And that keeps plaque from building up and causing problems.

To get the biggest gum-saving bang for your buck, buy xylitol in the form of sugar-free chewing gum. Not only will you get the xylitol effect, but chewing the gum triggers saliva production, which makes your mouth less acidic and washes away food and bacteria. Some gums don't have enough of this additive to block mouth bacteria, so look for 100 percent sweetening with xylitol on the label. Just don't overdo it, since too much of this good thing can cause diarrhea.

Natural solutions get nod from science

Dental floss dates back to prehistoric man. Early forms of the toothbrush have been around since 3000 BC. The Chinese used toothpaste in 500 BC. Not everything that is old is out-of-date. But today, modern dentistry helps us sort the crackpot remedies from those that really work.

Soothe painful gums with a teabag. People used to hold a warm, wet teabag next to a painful tooth to make it feel better. If it's green tea in that bag, experts say try it on your sore gums. Certain natural chemicals in green tea, called polyphenols, keep mouth bacteria from producing waste that damages your gums. Green tea extract is also added to some toothpaste.

Add tea tree oil to your brushing routine. This natural antiseptic is known to kill bacteria, and it's especially tough on the kind that causes gum disease. People with gingivitis noticed their symptoms improved after they rubbed tea tree gel on their gums. Certain toothpastes already contain tea tree oil, or you can add it yourself. Place one or two drops of the oil on top of your regular toothpaste, then brush. As with toothpaste, don't swallow.

Homespun remedies

Salt and sage make soothing mouthwash

Brew up a batch of fresh-tasting mouthwash with old-time ingredients. Steep 3 teaspoons of sage leaves in a cup of boiling water for 15 minutes, strain, then mix in 2 teaspoons of sea salt. Store this rinse in the refrigerator, and use it twice a day to help keep your gums healthy. Sage kills bacteria in your mouth, and sea salt is thought to fight inflammation.

Chew on some pine bark. Pycnogenol, a natural chemical from the bark of certain pine trees, works like other antioxidants to mop up cellular waste products and slow the effects of aging. In a two-week study, people chewed gum with added pycnogenol six times a day for a minimum of 15 minutes each – a total daily dose of 30 milligrams. Researchers checked their mouths before and after the study and found the pycnogenol helped clear up gum bleeding and reduced plaque formation. You may not find this gum for sale, but see if pycnogenol supplements help.

Traditional chewing stick gets the job done

Thousands of years before man developed the modern toothbrush, he chewed on sticks to clean his teeth. The miswak, or siwak, is a type of chewing stick still used in Africa and Asia – and credited with the good condition of teeth in those countries. Natives chew on a small stick to flatten it and form a brush on one end, then use the shaped stick to brush their teeth, remove food from between teeth, and scrape their tongues. Experts think the particular plants they fashion into chewing sticks contain natural chemicals that fight bacteria and help in other ways.

Now scientists have shown, in the hands of an experienced user, a miswak can clean teeth and gums as well as a toothbrush. Studies out of the Sudan, Saudi Arabia, and Ghana found chewing sticks:

- lessened gum bleeding.
- reduced plaque and mouth bacteria.
- neutralized harmful, plaque-causing acids in saliva.

You can get some of the benefits of the traditional chewing stick by chewing on a toothpick. For a fancier version, try the flavored and carefully shaped plaque-removing products like Johnson & Johnson's Stim-U-Dent or DenTek Super Pik. Remember, though, dentists aren't ready to tell you to toss out your toothbrush and toothpaste.

Hay Fever

Take a breather from pollen misery

Ahh, the good old days, when the word "allergy" didn't exist. Hard to imagine, but it wasn't until the early 1900s – when allergic diseases like hay fever, asthma, eczema, and food allergies exploded in the world's population – that it even became necessary to name this condition. In fact, 200 years ago, hay fever was a rare disorder. Now, it's the fourth most common chronic disease in the United States.

If you've inherited the super-sensitive immune system of an allergy sufferer, you know it overreacts to normally harmless substances – like pollen. Your body releases histamines when it shouldn't, and your blood vessels dilate and your tissues swell. You produce more mucus than normal and start sneezing, wheezing, sniffling, tearing, and itching.

According to folklore, if you want allergy relief you can wait for the night of a new moon, then walk barefoot in the dewy grass. Or you could cut a willow switch, throw it in the loft of your barn, and wait for it to dry.

But common sense says avoiding the problem should be your first line of defense. That means keeping allergens in your home and workplace to a minimum. So before you do anything else, try these simple tricks that will cut back on the number of allergens you encounter and help keep the air in your home fresh.

- Keep windows closed and stay inside as much as possible, especially from sunrise to 10 in the morning when pollen count is highest.

- Wear a mask to cover your mouth and nose when you garden or clean.
- Change clothes and take a shower after being outdoors to remove any pollen from your skin and hair.
- Use wet products to clean your house whenever possible. These trap pollen and other allergens that have made their way indoors.

If you're still suffering from a miserable allergy season, here are some other ideas to help you feel better.

Green tea: grass-roots allergy defense

Put away those tissues and breathe your way through allergy season. Just keep a cup of green tea close at hand. A powerful antioxidant in this ancient leaf may stop your body from reacting to allergens, like dust or pollen. Experts believe it also prevents the release of histamine, that pesky natural chemical behind your runny nose and itchy eyes. Because boiling water destroys some of the antioxidants in green tea, steep it in water that is hot, not boiling, for about three minutes. Drink it before it cools and the tea turns dark brown – a sign the antioxidants are no longer active.

Honey halts a pollen invasion

Springtime may mean pollen, but it also means flowers, bees, and honey. That's good news if you, like many people, believe local honey, made from local flowers, is full of local pollen, which might relieve your symptoms. By eating a daily tablespoon of locally produced, raw honey, you're introducing a small amount of pollen into your body. Later, when you breathe in that same pollen, your immune system may not overreact to it. See if this strategy works for you. Buy locally collected honey at your nearby farmer's market or health food store. Or, as some experts recommend, chew a small square of beeswax or honeycomb for about 10 to 15 minutes. Swallow the honey, but not the wax.

MythBuster: To stifle or to sneeze?

Holding in a sneeze may seem like polite behavior, but are you doing your body more harm than good? No one can argue the social consequences of spraying your neighbor every time your nose tickles, but experts say suppressing a sneeze keeps germs and irritants inside your body, when the whole purpose of a sneeze is to get rid of them. It's even possible – not likely, but possible – you could burst an eardrum from all that bottled-up pressure. The best course of action is to sneeze with your nose and mouth open, but covered with a tissue.

Humming: a "hum"-dinger of a congestion cure

A stuffy nose is one of the most uncomfortable symptoms of hay fever. Yet, your favorite tune could bring you relief – if you hum it. Humming causes sound waves to bounce around in your sinus cavities, possibly shaking things up enough to improve air flow and clear out mucus. There's also a more technical theory that includes nitric oxide and blood vessels and your immune system, but not much of that has been proven. Humming, at the very least, can be a happy, relaxing, and free pastime. So, all together now … hmmmmmm.

Nasal rinse blows allergens away

Think about the plumbing in your house. When it gets clogged, you do your best to flush out the pipes. The same is true when you're stuffed up with seasonal allergies. Step one is to flush out your nose. Not only will you feel better without excess mucus and allergens trapped in there, but any nasal medication will have a better chance of getting where it needs to go.

Start with clean hands and mix one-half teaspoon of uniodized salt – iodized salt can be irritating over time – and a pinch of baking soda into 8 ounces of warm water. Use a bulb syringe, sinus rinse bottle, or a "neti" pot, which you'll find at most drugstores. Squeeze, or pour, the saline solution into one nostril at a time, and then blow your nose gently. Repeat with the other nostril. Clean your equipment thoroughly after each use with hot water, then rubbing alcohol.

Vitamin C: a powerful antihistamine

Natural antihistamines allow your body to control how much histamine your white blood cells release. They can even neutralize the histamine that slips through. Multi-talented vitamin C also happens to be a natural antihistamine. The more you have circulating through your body, the lower your chances of suffering from allergies. That means eating C-rich foods regularly keeps you primed to fight off a hay fever attack. Foods that boost your C power include kiwis, red and green peppers, broccoli, cabbage, citrus fruits, berries, and guavas. But you can also take a supplement. Experts say you can safely take up to 1 gram of vitamin C a day.

Omega-3s end sinus distress

It just makes sense. Foods that have anti-inflammatory powers should help you through a condition that's all about inflammation. After all, aren't your sinuses, eyes, and throat red, swollen, and painful when you're suffering with hay fever? Omega-3 fatty acids reduce the number of enzymes in your body that promote inflammation. Good sources of this helpful fat are flaxseed; walnuts; wheat germ; dark, leafy green vegetables; and cold-water fish, like salmon, mackerel, and herring.

Spicy foods break up the bottleneck

Turn up the heat in your kitchen and you just might turn down your hay fever symptoms. Start cooking with hot, spicy ingredients, which can thin your mucus. Once your nose gets running, you'll

Watch out for herbal reactions

Soothing herbal teas have long been a remedy for allergy symptoms. Ginkgo, peppermint, fenugreek, and anise are just a few of the brews recommended by folk healers. Just remember, not all herbs will relieve the symptoms of pollen allergies. Many contain leaves or pollen that can trigger an allergic reaction. Echinacea tea, for example, is a common homespun remedy for a cold, so if you have a stuffy head from seasonal allergies, you might think this would be a safe choice. But echinacea tea has produced even worse allergic symptoms in many people. Choose your herbal remedies with care and start using them slowly so you can back off at the first sign of an allergic reaction.

find it easier to clear out your nasal passages and breathe again. So bring out the cayenne pepper, onion, ginger, fenugreek, and garlic. Or try horseradish, another spicy food guaranteed to blast open clogged sinuses. Mix a tablespoon of horseradish with a bit of honey, and not only will the sweet cut the heat, you'll be combining two allergy busters into one.

Steam unstuffs a stuffy nose

Inhaling vapors is as old as fire. People once gathered round the flames and breathed in steam from herbal brews to treat a variety of illnesses. Today, we're only slightly more sophisticated in this hay fever remedy. Basically, you combine boiling water with fresh or dried herbs, leaves, or essential oils, and breathe in the vapors through your nose. Draping a large towel over your head and the bowl creates a kind of tent that concentrates the benefits. Here are three ways to unblock your congestion.

- Place one-half ounce of ground thyme into a container with a lid and pour in two cups of boiling water. Close the container tightly and let this cool for about 30 minutes. Throughout the day, take the lid off and breathe deeply of the vapors.

- Boil eucalyptus leaves in a large pot, turn off the heat, and breathe in the steam.
- Pour one quart of boiling water into a large bowl containing either one-fourth ounce of peppermint leaves or two or three drops of peppermint essential oil. Inhale the steam for 10 to 15 minutes.

Quercetin quiets histamine

Quercetin, a natural chemical found in many foods, is also a natural antihistamine, regulating the membranes in your body that release histamine. You'll find it in apples, onions, citrus fruits, and buckwheat. There's quite a controversy over whether you can get enough quercetin from foods to ease you through allergy season. Even though supplements are available, some experts wonder whether taking plant chemicals out of their original "package" allows them to do the same job. If you decide to try quercetin supplements, the recommended dosage ranges from 250 to 600 milligrams, three times daily.

Herbal butterbur eases breathing

Want the benefits of an antihistamine without the drowsiness? A natural extract may be your answer. Butterbur, a plant native to Europe, Asia, and parts of North America, has been used in folk medicine for centuries. An extract from the leaves is believed to control the chemicals in your body that produce inflammation. Less inflammation means less stuffiness. Studies of the herbal supplement showed good results when volunteers took three tablets a day for two weeks. However, experts say to make sure the extract you take has had certain potentially dangerous chemicals – called pyrrolizidine alkaloids – removed. And talk to your doctor before you mix an alternative treatment like this with a traditional antihistamine.

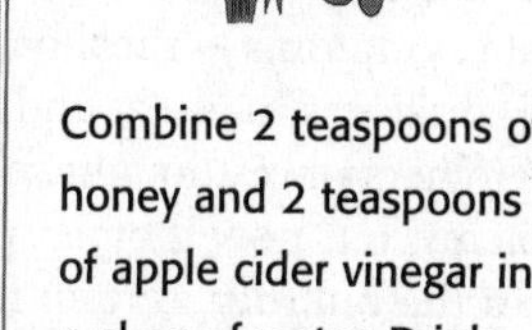

Combine 2 teaspoons of honey and 2 teaspoons of apple cider vinegar in a glass of water. Drink twice a day during hay fever season.

Headaches

Wise ways to head off head pain

You're keeping some pretty famous company if you battle serious headaches. Julius Caesar, Napoleon, and Elvis Presley all struggled with them. In fact, 40 percent of people have headaches severe enough to interfere with daily living. Fortunately, we've come a long way in headache treatment since bloodletting was used a few centuries ago. Today's experts know more about which cures work and why.

One key to the right remedy is knowing what kind of headache you have. Over 300 health conditions can cause head pain, from the benign – simple eyestrain – to the truly serious – a blood clot in the brain, for example. That's why it's important to see your general health care provider, eye doctor, and dentist for regular checkups. But if your pain isn't a symptom of another illness, you probably have one of the "Big Three" – a migraine headache, a tension headache, or a cluster headache.

Migraine headaches. You might mistake a migraine for a sinus or tension headache, but an experienced doctor should recognize the telltale symptoms – throbbing pain usually on one side of your head, dizziness, nausea, and high sensitivity to light or sound. Researchers once thought migraines stemmed from blood vessel problems, but now they suspect faulty brain chemistry. If you are one of the unlucky, certain foods, activities, or events may trigger migraines, even though no one is certain why. Some experts blame hyperactive brain cells, but inflammation, chemical imbalances, an agitated head nerve, blood flow problems, and a temporary plunge in brain activity may also contribute. The good news is if you understand your triggers, you may eventually help ease or prevent migraines. Here's the first place to start.

- Keep a headache diary. After each migraine, add an entry describing how long it lasted and its severity. Then list the times you went to bed and woke up that day plus all food, drinks, and medication you had during the 24 hours before the attack. Show the diary to your doctor so she can check for a pattern.
- Exercise regularly. Aerobic exercise like brisk walking and bike riding may help prevent migraines. But warm up first because sudden exertion can trigger an attack.
- Watch your weight. If you are overweight or obese, you are more likely to suffer from chronic migraines.

Tension headaches. These are the most common type of headache, and are characterized by a tight feeling of high-pressure pain on both sides of your head. Emotional stress and muscle tension in your shoulders, head, and neck are the most famed causes. But nutrient shortages and chemical imbalances may also play a part.

To help ease and prevent tension headaches, take an occasional nonsteroidal anti-inflammatory medication like ibuprofen or follow these tips to steer clear of the next headache.

- Avoid stressful events or reduce stress with relaxation exercises.
- Keep regular sleeping and eating schedules.
- Avoid eyestrain.

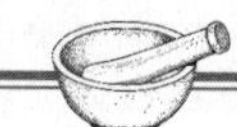

Breathing exercises that reduce stress may counteract the muscle tightness and blood flow problems that play a role in some headaches. Try this one from time to time. Rest one hand on your stomach. Take a slow, deep breath while counting from one to four. Then count down from four to one as you breathe out.

Homespun remedies

Press your pain away

This simple trick from an acupressure expert may ease your tension or migraine headache. Place the hand you write with on a flat surface. Find the tenderest spot on the web between your thumb and first finger and press there for one minute. Then lie down for 15 minutes.

- Improve your posture.
- Watch your weight.
- Be wary of intense physical activity.

Cluster headaches. These tend to occur in a pattern – like the same time every day, often at night – and they usually bring sudden, excruciating pain behind one eye. Experts think cluster headaches may be caused by an irregularity in your hypothalamus, the section of your brain that helps control your body's natural sleep/wake cycle. It also regulates some of your brain's chemical messengers like melatonin and serotonin.

Here's how to avoid future cluster headaches.

- Limit or avoid alcohol.
- Reduce stress.
- Avoid foods, like processed meats, that contain the preservatives sodium nitrate or sodium nitrite.
- Get on a regular sleep cycle.
- Avoid becoming overheated and try sleeping in a cool bedroom.
- Avoid smoking, especially during the days or weeks when headaches occur.

Inflammation-fighters defy migraines

Oncoming migraines are a little like a soufflé recipe. Forget one ingredient and the whole dish collapses. Two particular supplements could collapse a migraine before it starts by interfering with a key ingredient – inflammation.

Glucosamine. Its additional healing powers were discovered quite by accident. Several people reported fewer migraine headaches while taking glucosamine for osteoarthritis. Then, a small Canadian study confirmed glucosamine had a noticeable effect on the number and severity of migraines after only six weeks. Just remember, glucosamine may not be safe if you have shellfish allergies, kidney problems, asthma, diabetes, or several other conditions. It may also interact with some drugs, so talk to your doctor before you use it. If she approves, you may take up to 1,500 milligrams a day.

12 top migraine triggers

Some foods or events can trigger that head-splitting pain. Yours may be different, but try avoiding these common triggers and you might avoid the pain – stress, too much or too little sleep, abrupt weather changes, travel motion, low blood sugar, and bright lights. In addition, many migraine sufferers find certain foods, like chocolate, will trigger an attack. Here are some food additives, both natural and artificial, that might be behind the trouble.

- sulfites in wine and dried fruit
- tannins in apple juice, tea, coffee, and red wine
- monosodium glutamate (MSG) in some Chinese food
- nitrates in processed meats
- artificial sweeteners like aspartame

Butterbur. If glucosamine isn't for you, consider the herbal extract, butterbur. Used as a remedy for plague in the Middle Ages, today's research suggests it contains inflammation-fighting compounds called petasin and isopetasin. When doctors ordered daily butterbur doses of 150 milligrams for people who had at least two migraines a month, the number of migraines during the four months of treatment dropped by nearly half.

Don't buy supplements or teas containing unprocessed butterbur. It's toxic. Instead, choose the brand Petadolex. This widely tested butterbur extract has been purified of toxins and is the only product herbal experts consider reliably safe and effective.

Soothing oils dissolve tension

Try this on your next tension headache. Add two drops of peppermint oil or eucalyptus oil to 8 ounces of water. Soak a washcloth in the mixture, wring it out, and hold the cloth against your head until the pain melts away. Or try mixing one teaspoon of peppermint oil with nine teaspoons of rubbing alcohol. Dampen a cotton ball in this blend, make sure it won't drip into your eyes, and then dab it on your bare forehead. Repeat in 15 minutes. A German study found this to be as effective in reducing head pain as taking 1,000 milligrams of acetaminophen. Research suggests both these oils may help relax your muscles and your mind.

Coffee: ancient cure or grounds for concern?

The power of coffee was discovered over a thousand years ago, folklore says. It happened when an Ethiopian goatherd noticed his goats became more energetic after eating the "berries" on a coffee bush. Once he tried a few himself, coffee was on its way to stardom. Of course, it's the caffeine that makes coffee so appealing. This natural stimulant travels from your stomach, through your blood, to your brain, where it not only causes your nerve cells to speed up but also constricts your brain's blood vessels. And that explains a recent study, which found the caffeine in two and a half cups of coffee treated a tension headache, even without painkillers.

Thaw the brain freeze

You ate your ice cream cone in a hurry because it was melting. And now your head hurts with a vengeance. Fortunately, the pain should fade in a minute or two. But the next time you have a chilly treat, warm the frozen stuff in the front of your mouth for a few seconds before swallowing.

But don't reach for that jumbo-size cup of java just yet. The tannins in coffee can be a migraine trigger for some people and caffeine, itself, can bring on recurring headaches. In fact, even caffeine withdrawal may cause headaches. So, if you drink a lot of coffee, tea, colas, or energy drinks daily, gradually cut back to two drinks a day to see if your headaches get better.

What's more, many pain and headache medications contain caffeine because it makes the drugs more effective. But drugs that contain caffeine are more likely to cause headaches if you take them more than three days each week – these are called medication-overuse headaches. Ask your doctor how you can safely switch to a caffeine-free drug.

Spunky spice derails migraines

The same spice that flavors scrumptious gingersnaps and gingerbread might help you dodge your next migraine. That's what a Danish woman discovered when her doctors suggested she try ginger. At the first hint of migraine, she mixed 500 to 600 milligrams of powdered ginger in plain water and drank it – and began feeling better within 30 minutes. As she added more ginger to her daily diet, her migraines became less severe and she had fewer of them.

Ginger acts in much the same way as nonsteroidal anti-inflammatory drugs (NSAIDs) like naproxen (Alleve, Naprosyn), ibuprofen (Motrin), and indomethacin (Indocin). They all reduce your body's levels of prostaglandins, natural chemicals that, among other things, are responsible for pain and inflammation. In addition, ginger may banish the nausea that comes with migraines.

Ginger

If you'd like to try ginger, ask your doctor first. Large doses of ginger may irritate your stomach, interact with insulin or antacids, or increase the effect of blood-thinning medications like aspirin and warfarin. Ginger can also be unsafe if you have gallbladder disease or upcoming surgery. But if your doctor gives the all-clear, add this spice to your diet gradually until you reach one-half to one teaspoon daily. Try it in stir-fries, carrot dishes, marinades, stews, sauces, sweet potatoes, or desserts. You can also make a tea by steeping several slices of raw ginger in hot water for 10 to 15 minutes. If ginger causes burping or burning in your throat, consider ginger capsules instead.

Melatonin: new hope for headaches

The same hormone that regulates your sleeping and waking may play a part in migraines and cluster headaches. It's a fact – migraine sufferers tend to be low in melatonin. Some experts blame this on an irregularity of the pineal gland at the base of your brain, where this important hormone is produced. Fortunately, early research suggests three months on a 3-milligram supplement of melatonin can lead to fewer migraines.

In addition, people with cluster headaches have low levels of this hormone, particularly at night. A small Italian study found that half the people who took a 10-milligram supplement of melatonin every evening began having fewer cluster headache attacks after five days.

If you'd like to try melatonin, be aware that you must avoid caffeine and alcohol while taking it. What's more, melatonin may interact with over-the-counter and prescription medicines as well as vitamin B12. Check with your doctor before you try melatonin because it isn't safe for everyone, especially in the large doses used in the studies.

When head pain spells danger

Even if you're already being treated for headaches, the American Council for Headache Education (ACHE) says to contact your doctor if you experience any of the following symptoms – you may have a more serious problem.

- three or more headaches weekly
- a need for regular and stronger pain relievers
- a headache that worsens and won't go away
- a headache with fever, shortness of breath, a stiff neck, dizziness, numbness, tingling, slurred speech, confusion, or severe vomiting
- headaches that began only after turning 50
- a headache triggered by coughing or exertion

Feverfew means fewer migraines

It may look like just another roadside flower, but feverfew is actually the most studied herb for headaches. And much of that research says take it and you'll get fewer migraines.

Like butterbur, feverfew fights the inflammation that can rev up a migraine, but feverfew goes one step further by keeping platelets in your blood from sticking together. That may help prevent a chain reaction affecting blood flow and migraine pain.

Experts recommend anywhere from 50 to 250 milligrams of a dried leaf product daily to prevent migraines, but an extract called MIG-99 has been successful, too. Just remember, feverfew may interact with some medications, so don't try it before getting your doctor's approval. If you experience mouth ulcers or stomach discomfort from this herb, don't stop taking it suddenly – you could experience withdrawal symptoms like rebound headaches. Instead, taper off gradually.

Hearing problems

Solutions that will cheer your ears

Did you hear the joke about the rooster and the rhino? Probably not, if you're hard of hearing. Aside from missing out on good jokes, hearing problems can make you feel cut off from the rest of the world, even from your family.

One in three people over age 60 has trouble hearing, as do half of people over the age of 85. Deafness isn't the only problem. Tinnitus – a ringing, roaring, or buzzing in your ears – afflicts about one in seven Americans. At best, it's annoying. At worst, it's incapacitating.

When sound enters your ear, it sets off a chain reaction. It makes your eardrum vibrate which, in turn, causes three tiny bones called the ossicles to vibrate. The ossicles send the vibrations into your cochlea, a snail-shaped chamber in your inner ear.

The cochlea is filled with fluid and tiny cells shaped like hairs. When sound vibrations move through the fluid, the waves shake the tops of these hairs, creating electrical impulses. Nerves carry these impulses from your ear to your brain, which interprets them as sounds. Different sound vibrations move the hairs differently, so your brain can tell words and other sounds apart.

Aging, loud noises, health problems, and even some medications can damage the delicate structures in your ear, leading to hearing loss, tinnitus, or both. Some risk factors you can't control, like family history. Others, like these, you can.

Kick those butts. Long-term smoking increases your risks for tinnitus and permanent, noise-related hearing damage. So quit now, while you're ahead. If you need help, talk with your doctor.

Cover your ears. Loud noise can also lead to hearing loss and tinnitus. Protect your hearing with earplugs or safety earmuffs while doing loud activities, like mowing the lawn. And keep the volume reasonable when you listen to music or television, especially if you use earphones.

Treat other conditions. Circulatory problems from heart disease, high blood pressure, and diabetes restrict the blood supply to your ears, which can harm hearing and worsen tinnitus. Controlling these health problems can help. Treating insomnia, anxiety, depression, and temporomandibular disorder (TMD) could also improve tinnitus.

Get outside help. Devices such as hearing aids and cochlear implants can greatly improve your hearing, plus help suppress tinnitus. Getting a hearing aid that fits and works well may take some trial and error. Don't give up. A hearing specialist, such as an audiologist, can help you find the right device.

Noise: how loud is too loud?

When the Edmonton Oilers played for the Stanley Cup in 2006, researchers measured noise levels in the hockey arena. During a three-hour match, audience and players not wearing hearing protection endured 81 times more sound than is safe. Simply wearing cheap foam earplugs during the game would have cut noise levels enough to prevent hearing damage.

Most people recover from short-term hearing loss, but the damage can accumulate over time. Even one-time loud sounds can permanently hurt your ears. Anything softer than 80 decibels (dB) is considered safe. You can tolerate louder noises for short periods of time, but the louder the noise, the less time you should spend around it. Check this list of common sounds and their loudness, and wear earplugs or earmuffs during noisy activities.

- whisper, quiet library (30 dB)
- hum from refrigerator (40 dB)
- normal conversation, sewing machine (60 dB)
- heavy city traffic (85 dB)
- lawnmower (90 dB)
- wood shop or snowmobile (100 dB)
- chain saw, rock concert (110 dB)
- car horn (115 dB)
- ambulance siren (120 dB)

Warm water melts away earwax

Hearing problems? You might have too much earwax, or you might be cleaning it out the wrong way. Earwax can become packed down inside your ear canal, causing hearing loss, pain, dizziness, and vertigo, as well as increasing your risk for an ear infection. It could even be causing tinnitus in some of the 1 million Americans who complain of ringing in their ears.

Cleaning your ears improperly with cotton swabs contributes to earwax buildup. The wax forms inside your ear canal. Your jaw muscles gradually help move it toward your outer ear. When you insert a cotton swab in your ear canal, you may get a little soft earwax on the end, but you pack down the solid wax in your canal. Doing this enough times can make it hard and impacted, like a wax earplug.

For most people, washing your outer ear daily with a soapy washcloth is all you need to keep your ears clean. But if you struggle with earwax buildup, there's a good chance you can remove it yourself with these effortless solutions. These easy home remedies are available at any drugstore without a prescription.

For each of the following methods, you'll need an ear bulb syringe filled with warm water to rinse out your ear canals. The best way to do it – insert the tip just inside your ear canal. Grab the top of your ear, and pull up and back. Aim for the roof of your ear canal, and very gently squeeze the bulb. Stand over the sink to catch any drips. Be careful not to squeeze the bulb too hard, since excessive water pressure can damage your eardrum. Now you're ready to choose a remedy.

Water. Fill your ear canal with warm water, then use a wet cotton ball to block the canal opening. Leave the water in for 15 minutes. Remove the cotton, fill the bulb syringe with lukewarm water, and rinse out your ear canal.

Oil. Heat a small amount of mineral or vegetable oil to body temperature by placing the bottle in a pan of warm, not hot, water for several minutes. Put a drop or two of the oil in your ear canal, and cover the opening with a cotton ball. Wait 10 to 15 minutes for the oil to soften the wax, then rinse with warm water using the bulb syringe.

Carbamide peroxide. Look for over-the-counter earwax removers made with carbamide peroxide. It foams gently like the peroxide you dab on cuts, loosening hardened earwax so you can safely rinse it out. Follow the directions carefully for each product.

Don't try to remove earwax yourself if you notice any drainage or discharge from your ear or have pain, irritation, or a rash in your

An earful about earwax

Earwax isn't all bad. In fact, it's mostly good. It coats your ear canal, capturing dirt, bugs, and other foreign objects before they reach the delicate structures inside your ears. It also boasts antibacterial properties, which help prevent ear infections.

ear. Instead, see your doctor. These symptoms could signal a more serious problem.

Background sounds quiet the clamor

Avoiding total quiet is one of the most important things you can do to silence tinnitus. Quiet makes the ringing in your ears seem louder – loud enough to drive you crazy. Background noise helps cover up the din by making it less noticeable.

Masking is a key treatment for tinnitus and helps about 15 percent of people. You don't even need expensive equipment. The soft buzz of a table fan or any of these options could do the trick.

☛ Tune the FM dial on your radio to the static between stations if you have trouble sleeping or whenever your house is quiet.

Beware drugs that hurt your hearing

Some medications are ototoxic, meaning they can damage your hearing, leading to hearing loss or tinnitus. Aspirin, for instance, can trigger both problems, while hormone replacement therapy (HRT) combining estrogen and progesterone may increase your risk of hearing loss. The following drugs, in particular, can cause hearing loss or tinnitus.

- nonsteroidal anti-inflammatory drugs (NSAIDs) (ibuprofen, naproxen)
- aminoglycoside antibiotics, such as gentamicin (Garamycin, G-Mycin, Jenamicin)
- cisplatin (Platinol, Platinol-AQ)
- vancomycin (Vancocin)
- loop diuretics, such as furosemide (Lasix)
- valproic acid (divalproex sodium, valproate sodium, Depakene, Depakote)
- quinine in high doses (Quinamm, Quiphile)

- Play relaxing music on your stereo or turn on your TV as background noise.
- Invest in an inexpensive sound generator that mimics the ocean, rain, or white noise. Retailers, like Target, sell them for around $25. Some hook up to a special pillow with speakers inside so the noise doesn't disturb your family.
- Look for devices specifically made to mask tinnitus. Some fit in your ear, like a hearing aid.
- Get fitted for a hearing aid if you have hearing loss. The ringing in your ears can seem loud simply because you can't hear outside noise. You can also buy hearing aids that include a tinnitus masker.

6 simple ways to enhance your hearing

Don't let hearing loss keep you from the activities and people you love. These simple adjustments can help you live a full life.

- Let people, including friends and family, know you have trouble hearing.
- Ask people to face you when they speak. Reading their lips and facial expressions can help you understand what they say.
- Visit noisy places, like restaurants, during the quieter, off-peak hours so you can better hear conversation.
- Request a booth at restaurants to block out background noise, and ask to be seated away from loud areas, like the kitchen or a band playing music.
- Take a class in lip reading through an "aural rehabilitation" program.
- Turn off the radio or TV if you aren't paying attention to it. You're more likely to hear important sounds, like the doorbell and telephone.

HEART ATTACK

Tips to keep your ticker ticking

Your heart never takes a vacation. It works constantly to pump blood throughout your body. But, like your other organs, your heart needs blood, too. Oxygen-rich blood returns to your heart through the coronary arteries. Everything runs smoothly until one of your coronary arteries becomes blocked. Then your hard-working heart may earn an instant – and permanent – vacation. That's what happens when you have a heart attack, the leading cause of death in the United States.

Heart attacks may strike instantly, but they are years in the making. Atherosclerosis, or the buildup of plaque on your artery walls, is usually to blame. Plaque can either build up until it completely blocks an artery, or it can rupture or crack, leading to a blood clot. This cuts off the blood supply to the myocardium, the muscular layer of the heart wall that helps the heart pump. Without the oxygen it needs, the heart muscle will die.

A heart attack – also known as a myocardial infarction – can strike anyone, but older people and blacks are at greater risk. Other risk factors include a sedentary lifestyle, obesity, smoking, high blood pressure, high cholesterol, and a family history of heart attacks. Before age 50, men are more likely to have a heart attack than women – but, after menopause, women's risk increases as their levels of estrogen decrease.

Be on the lookout. Heart attacks announce themselves in several ways. The most common sign of a heart attack is crushing pain in your chest, which can radiate to your arms – especially your left arm, shoulders, neck, jaw, back, or abdomen. You may also feel a sense of fullness, squeezing, or pressure in your chest. However, nearly half of all women and a third of all men feel no chest pain or discomfort at all during a heart attack. Often, women suffer from unusual fatigue, sleep disturbances, and shortness of breath for about a month before the heart attack. Other signs of a heart attack include profuse sweating, lightheadedness, nausea, a feeling of heartburn, shortness of breath, dizziness, and fainting.

If you experience any of these symptoms, call 911 right away. You may also want to chew an aspirin, which stops blood clots from forming. Fast action can save your life and limit the damage to your heart.

Plan ahead. Of course, the best strategy is to prevent a heart attack in the first place. Keep your heart in tip-top shape with these simple tips.

- Eat a healthy diet low in saturated fat – found in foods like meat, butter, cheese, and whole milk – and rich in fruits, vegetables, and whole grains.
- Exercise regularly. Aim for 30 minutes of moderate exercise a day.
- Lose weight if you're overweight.
- Keep your blood pressure and cholesterol levels within a healthy range.
- Quit smoking.
- Drink alcohol in moderation, if at all. That means no more than two drinks a day for a man and one drink for a woman.

You may also want to ask your doctor about low-dose aspirin therapy. Taking an aspirin a day can help prevent heart attacks in men and in women over age 65. However, aspirin therapy is not for everyone. Aspirin increases the risk of stomach or intestinal bleeding and hemorrhagic stroke – dangers that may outweigh its benefits if you're not at high risk for a heart attack.

Keep reading to discover more ways to prevent or deal with a heart attack.

Mediterranean diet heals a broken heart

Look to the Mediterranean to help your heart. You don't need to visit Greece or Italy – just adopt the region's eating habits.

A recent Italian study found that staples of the Mediterranean diet help people live longer after a heart attack. Heart attack survivors who ate the most fish, fruit, raw and cooked vegetables, and olive oil cut their risk of death in half compared to those who ate the least of these heart-healthy foods. The Mediterranean diet also features plenty of canola oil, nuts, legumes, beans, and whole grains. Its tasty seasonings include garlic, onions, and herbs.

Here's a quick look at three important additions to a heart-healthy diet.

Fish. Rich in omega-3 fatty acids, fish protects your heart in many ways. Several studies show that eating fish slashes your risk of heart disease or sudden death from a heart attack or stroke. Exactly how fish helps remains unclear, but fish oil can counteract irregular heartbeats, lower blood pressure and triglycerides, and fight inflammation – all good defenses against heart attacks. Aim for at least two fatty fish meals a week. Tuna, salmon, herring, mackerel, sardines, and trout are your best choices.

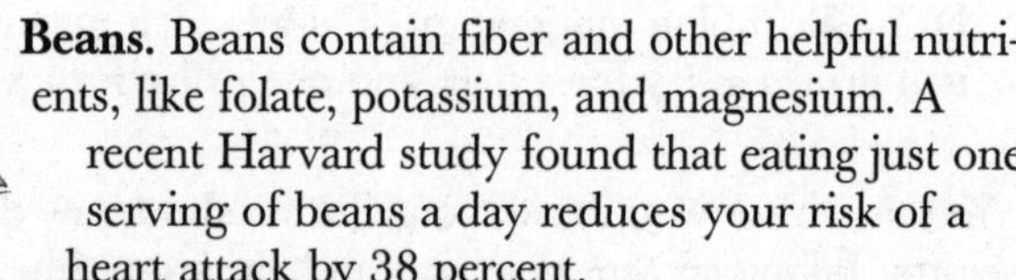

Beans. Beans contain fiber and other helpful nutrients, like folate, potassium, and magnesium. A recent Harvard study found that eating just one serving of beans a day reduces your risk of a heart attack by 38 percent.

Water. Make sure to drink plenty of water. Drinking five or more glasses of water a day can dramatically reduce your risk of a fatal heart attack.

You might also want to consider taking a multivitamin every day. While it's usually better to get your nutrients from food rather than pills, Swedish researchers discovered that taking a multivitamin supplement lowers the risk of a heart attack in both men (21 percent) and women (34 percent).

Coffee and tea impact heart attack risk

That morning cup of coffee really perks you up. Unfortunately, your risk of having a heart attack may go up, too. Several studies have found links between coffee and heart attacks. How much coffee you drink, how often you drink it, how you prepare it, and how your body metabolizes it all have an impact on your heart.

In a Finnish study, men who drank three-and-a-half cups of coffee or more had a 43-percent greater risk of heart attack than those who drank less. Another study found that those who drank coffee only occasionally were at greater risk than heavy coffee drinkers.

Boiled coffee, the kind you make in a French press, poses more of a threat than filtered coffee. A recent study determined that people

Holidays bring unwanted surprise

Family, friends, presents, and food all go hand-in-hand with the holiday season. Unfortunately, so do heart attacks. Whether it's because of the cold winter weather, the added stress, or delays in seeking treatment, heart-related deaths increase by more than 4 percent around Christmas and New Year's. The tendency to overeat during the holidays can also play a role. Studies show eating an unusually large meal dramatically raises your risk of a heart attack. Play it safe around the holidays. Keep your portions under control, stick to your exercise routine, avoid last-minute holiday shopping and other stressful situations, and seek help immediately if you experience heart attack symptoms.

who metabolize coffee slowly have a much greater risk of a heart attack than those who metabolize it quickly. To be safe, limit yourself to one or two cups of coffee a day. Avoid coffee if it leaves you feeling weak or lightheaded or gives you a racing pulse or chest pain.

You could also switch to tea. A Dutch study of older men and women found that tea drinkers had a lower risk of heart attack – especially a fatal heart attack – than people who don't drink tea. Even if you do have a heart attack, drinking tea may help you live longer afterward.

Sweet news for chocolate lovers

Snacking on chocolate can help your heart. A recent study found that chocolate helps prevent platelet clumping, similar to aspirin. That reduces the risk of blood clots – and heart attacks. Previous studies have identified several other heart-healthy properties of cocoa and chocolate, which are rich in flavonoids. These antioxidants may

MythBuster: Can coughing save your life?

During cardiac arrest, when your heart suddenly stops pumping, a few coughs might be the difference between life and death. Coughing helps pump blood through your body and to your brain so you don't lose consciousness before help arrives. At the first sign of trouble, cough forcefully every one to two seconds in sets of five coughs.

The American Heart Association does not endorse "cough CPR" or teach it as a technique in its CPR courses – not because it doesn't work, but because it only helps in rare instances. It's much more important to call 911 for emergency help at the first sign of a heart attack.

lower blood pressure, fight inflammation, and widen blood vessels by relaxing the muscles in their walls. But that doesn't mean you should pig out on candy bars. A little chocolate goes a long way. Just two tablespoons of dark chocolate a day should do the trick.

Peace and quiet protects your heart

Stress comes in many forms, and none of them is good for your heart. Road rage, traffic jams, noisy workplaces or living conditions, and high-pressure deadlines all increase your risk of having a heart attack. Being prone to anger, overworking – such as never taking a sick day, even when you're sick – and having a type A personality do not help, either. That's because your body responds to stressful situations by releasing hormones, like adrenaline, that boost your heart rate, raise your blood pressure, and can cause spasms in your coronary arteries.

Whenever stress gets hold of you, take a deep breath and relax. Finding healthy ways to cope with stress can help safeguard your heart. One study found that stress management techniques, including biofeedback and progressive muscle relaxation, lowered the risk of a heart attack or other heart event by 74 percent. Just taking a walk or chatting with family and friends can also help.

Pets tame heart problems

Your furry friend does more than just fetch or roll over. Pets also provide top-notch benefits to your heart. When in the company of their pets, people tend to have lower heart rates and blood pressure. They also respond better to stress. So it makes sense that after a heart attack, pet owners fare better than people without pets.

When considering a pet, remember to take into account the cost of food and veterinarian bills, plus the amount of care and attention the pet will need. For instance, a dog demands more time and energy than a cat. If you're renting, make sure your landlord allows pets before getting one.

HEARTBURN

Natural healers and helpers put out the fire

Heartburn will vanish if you attach a mushroom to the northern beam of your stable – according to an old folk remedy. Then again, if you don't have a stable, you may need something more practical and promising to fight the burn.

If you're wondering what causes heartburn, here's what's going on. Your stomach secretes hydrochloric acid and other juices to digest food, but it's supposed to keep the acid to itself. In fact, a valve, called the lower esophageal sphincter or LES, sits at the top of your stomach to make sure no acid escapes. It opens long enough to let food in but closes quickly before stomach acid can escape.

However, sometimes the LES relaxes when it shouldn't, allowing stomach acid into your esophagus. That's when you feel burning or pain in your chest or throat. You may even get a bitter taste in your mouth or feel hot liquid rising in your throat.

If heartburn only happens occasionally, it's usually harmless. But heartburn can be a sign of heart attack or GERD – gastroesophageal reflux disease. That's when heartburn may be serious and you should see your doctor. If your heartburn is accompanied by nausea, breathlessness, fainting, sweating, weakness, or shooting pain from your jaw to your arm, you might be having a heart attack. Call 911 for help.

If you get heartburn two times a week or more, you may have chronic heartburn or GERD. The word "reflux" refers to the times when acid splashes up into your esophagus. If reflux happens often enough, it can cause damage. Serious damage may lead to deadly cancer of the esophagus. Play it safe and see your doctor for help with frequent heartburn.

On the other hand, if your heartburn isn't severe or frequent and you have no heart attack symptoms, why pay for expensive drugs, tests, and procedures when you don't have to? Discover all the best natural healers here, and how to use them. Start with these fire fighters.

- Chew your food a little more. Chewing increases saliva, which neutralizes acid.
- Stop eating when you feel full. Overeating and large meals rev up acid production.
- Don't eat for at least two hours before bedtime, and don't lie down for at least two hours after eating. Your stomach needs time to empty out both food and acid. Singer Kenny Rogers says late night eating after concerts probably contributed to his heartburn problems.
- Lose some weight. It might be the most powerful lifestyle change you can make. That's because extra pounds squeeze your stomach area, loosening the LES and pushing acid into your esophagus.
- Wear clothes and belts that fit comfortably around your midsection. Tight clothes can also put pressure on your stomach area.

MythBuster: Does milk soothe your stomach?

Milk is often recommended as a stomach soother, but this Dr. Jekyll has a Mr. Hyde side. It lowers the pressure of the LES so stomach acid can sneak out and cause heartburn. On top of that, milk temporarily relieves heartburn, then increases stomach acid production later. Skip the milk. You might put out the flames before they start.

- Find a way to quit smoking. Smoking loosens the LES, boosts acid production, and decreases the saliva in your mouth. This not only encourages heartburn, it prevents saliva from sweeping acid out of your esophagus.
- Avoid heavy lifting and straining. When you lift something, your abdominal muscles contract and squeeze stomach acid into your esophagus.
- Learn to manage and reduce stress. Taking a walk, writing in a journal, watching a funny movie, or getting enough sleep can help.

2 ways chewing gum puts out the fire

A stick of chewing gum gives you fast heartburn relief – and it works in minutes. That's because chewing gum beats the burn in two ways.

First, it makes you swallow more often, which moves acid out of your esophagus and back into your stomach where it belongs. Second, chewing gum causes your mouth to make more saliva. Your spit doesn't just help dilute acid – it also contains acid-fighting compounds. In fact, researchers discovered that just a half hour of chewing gum right after a meal cuts acid in your esophagus for several hours. That fights heartburn and might even protect against damage from GERD.

Dodge heartburn drug dangers

Medicines like Tagamet or Prilosec could put you at risk for dementia, loss of balance, muscle weakness, incontinence, and moodiness. That's because these are consequences of vitamin B12 deficiency, a condition acid blocker drugs can cause. Taking an acid blocker for two years or longer may limit your ability to absorb enough B12 from food, but your doctor probably can't detect that deficiency with a routine blood test. Talk with her about whether your acid-blocking medicines could be causing a vitamin B12 deficiency and get her advice on whether a B12 supplement is right for you.

So start chewing gum right after a meal or anytime you feel heartburn coming on. But bypass the spearmint, peppermint, cinnamon, and ice flavors because these may trigger heartburn in some people. Instead, try the bubblegum flavor now available in both regular and sugarless gum. Chew the sugarless variety if you can because it helps prevent cavities. But stick with regular gum if artificial sweeteners, like sorbitol, give you gas, bloating, or diarrhea.

To score even more heartburn protection, drink water. Water rinses acid out of your esophagus and dilutes the acid in your stomach. Drink small amounts of water between meals throughout the day – just don't overdo it. Drinking too much at once could overstretch your stomach and make your heartburn worse.

Fennel tea: relief from a fragrant herb

In the Middle Ages, the Anglo-Saxons didn't have a corner drugstore so they turned to a feathery-leaved herb called fennel.

Tea made from sweet-scented fennel seeds contains a natural compound called anethole. This compound stimulates bile production and relieves spasms in your stomach and bowel muscles. Together, those changes help soothe heartburn and other digestive problems.

To make fennel seed tea, steep a teaspoon of seeds in a cup of boiled water for 15 minutes. Strain out the seeds and drink. If you need a stronger tea, crush the seeds before steeping. Enjoy this tea after or between meals two to three times daily.

But choose a different remedy if you're allergic to carrot, celery, or mugwort. You might be allergic to fennel, too.

Blocks end nightly distress

You don't have to take heartburn lying down. This trick works better than giving up certain foods. What's more, it's easy and research proves it works. Just put blocks under two bedposts to raise the head of your bed 6 inches higher. This keeps your stomach below your esophagus and lets gravity help fight your heartburn. If bedpost blocks aren't right for you, don't try extra pillows under your head. They raise your odds of heartburn and can give you a pain in the neck. Instead, get a sleeping wedge from a medical supply store, tuck it under your upper body, and enjoy sweet heartburn relief.

Baking soda: cheap cure or hidden hazard?

Baking soda might seem like the perfect answer to your heartburn problem, but new research shows it's not a good choice. Experts say when baking soda stops working, you'll get even more acid than you had before. And that's not the only reason to run from baking soda. Consider these.

- One-half teaspoon of Arm & Hammer Baking Soda contains a whopping 616 milligrams of sodium. That can be dangerous if you are on a sodium-restricted diet for high blood pressure or a heart condition.
- You might be tempted to take more every time heartburn comes roaring back if the first round of baking soda doesn't work. But taking too much could cause alkalosis, an imbalance in your body's acid-base levels. That can be extremely dangerous.
- Baking soda may also be dangerous to take if you feel too full after eating or drinking.

You might think baking powder is a safe alternative to baking soda, but that's not true. Although baking powder contains baking soda, it also includes ingredients that are harmful to take. Play it safe. Leave the baking soda and baking powder on the shelf and stick with safer remedies.

Diary ends pointless food restrictions

Some people say cinnamon, hot peppers, and ginger can cause heartburn, while others claim they help put out the flames. A recent discovery may help explain this paradox. Scientists now say eliminating foods doesn't help everyone who has GERD. What's

Nab a hidden trigger

Aspirin and other nonsteroidal anti-inflammatory drugs (NSAIDs) can increase your risk of developing GERD or make it worse if you already have it. These NSAIDS include some prescription painkillers, as well as over-the-counter drugs, like ibuprofen (Advil) and naproxen (Aleve). Acetaminophen (Tylenol) is a safe alternative. Other examples of potential fire starters include certain sedatives, antibiotics, iron pills, drugs for high blood pressure and angina, and osteoporosis medications, like Fosamax. Ask your doctor if any medicines you take might bring on GERD or make it worse. You may be able to switch to a safer alternative.

more, conflicting studies are making researchers question whether foods like chocolate and coffee cause heartburn.

You can cope with this confusion by starting a diary. Keep track of what you eat and when you have symptoms. You'll soon notice what foods trigger heartburn. Best of all, you'll be able to add old favorites back into your diet. Pay close attention to these foods.

- table salt and salted meats or fish
- coffee and tea – with caffeine and without, alcoholic beverages, and carbonated drinks
- foods that are greasy, fried, spicy, or high in saturated fat
- citrus fruits and juices – orange, lemon, lime, and grapefruit
- tomato products, including ketchup
- foods and drinks containing chocolate, peppermint, or spearmint
- cinnamon, cloves, ginger, pepper, onions, garlic, and vinegar

Hemorrhoids

Simple steps soothe the swelling

Few conditions are as embarrassing or uncomfortable as hemorrhoids. In a culture where almost anything goes, it's still a taboo topic. But a lot of people are hiding something, because about half the population has had them by age 50.

Hemorrhoids are nothing more than swollen veins, much like varicose veins in your legs. When the veins outside the anus swell, they are called external hemorrhoids. When veins inside your rectum swell, they are internal hemorrhoids – although sometimes these prolapse, or slip out through your anus. Internal hemorrhoids don't usually hurt, but the external ones can, especially if they develop a blood clot. These are called thrombosed external hemorrhoids. All types can bleed, and the external ones often itch.

Blame your parents, if you like, because hemorrhoids tend to run in families. Straining with constipation or diarrhea may trigger them, but, in truth, anything that puts pressure on these veins – an enlarged prostate, chronic cough, liver disease, or being very overweight – increases your risk. All is not lost, however. Experts say you can usually manage hemorrhoids with a few precautions.

Spend less time on the toilet. The only time your anus muscles really relax is when you sit on the toilet. This allows the veins in the area to fill with blood. The longer you sit, the longer those veins are under pressure.

Stay active. Since it hurts to sit, you might as well get up and move. Walking, exercising, and generally being active combat constipation by helping move stool through your bowels. And standing up rather than sitting down relieves pressure on your veins.

Avoid certain laxatives. Sure, constipation can worsen hemorrhoids, but so can diarrhea. Bulk-forming laxatives, such as Metamucil and Fiberall, are generally safe, but stay away from others unless your doctor says otherwise.

Over-the-counter pain relievers like aspirin, ibuprofen (Advil), and acetaminophen (Tylenol) can ease the pain of occasional flare-ups. Most hemorrhoids go away within a week or two, but see your doctor if yours last longer or if you see blood. You want to make sure the bleeding is caused by hemorrhoids and not a more serious problem, like colon cancer.

Bathroom habits beat the burn

Hemorrhoids can turn a simple trip to the bathroom into an ordeal. Take the sting out of staying regular with these time-tested tips.

- Head to the bathroom as soon as you feel the urge for a bowel movement.
- Prop your feet up a few inches on a footstool, phone book, or other object while sitting on the toilet. This position helps you pass stool with less strain.
- Wipe gently with wet toilet paper or moist towelettes, but don't wipe excessively.
- Take a quick shower if wiping hurts too much. Keeping the anal area clean reduces irritation, but don't use soap as it can aggravate hemorrhoids.
- After washing, dry the anal area well with either a soft cloth or a hair dryer on the lowest setting. Lingering moisture can cause irritation.

Sweet solution to hemorrhoid symptoms

This old-time remedy may shrink painful tissues in only a few minutes. Wet external hemorrhoids with water and sprinkle on a couple teaspoons of sugar. Dampen with a little more water.

High-fiber diet puts an end to hemorrhoids

Filling up on fiber will help fight those fiery hemorrhoids. A natural laxative, it combats the constipation that can lead to flare-ups by making stool soft, bulky, and easy to pass. In one study, people with internal, bleeding hemorrhoids took a daily dose of one rounded tablespoon of Metamucil powder, a psyllium laxative containing about 3 grams of fiber. After 40 days, they had less bleeding and fewer hemorrhoids.

More recently, experts reviewed seven studies and found fiber laxatives consistently relieved hemorrhoid symptoms, especially bleeding. Overall, people who took fiber laxatives were about half as likely to continue suffering with persistent hemorrhoids as those who didn't.

Supplements like Metamucil aren't the only way to get more fiber, though. Whole grains, wheat bran, and fresh fruits and vegetables are great natural sources. In fact, you can get the same amount of fiber used in the study by eating one apple, one cup of raw carrots, or one cup of Wheaties. What a delicious and healthy way to get that oh-so-important fiber. However you decide to get it, this advice will help you make the most of it.

- Aim to get a total of 25 to 30 grams of fiber daily.
- Start slowly and gradually increase your fiber intake to give your digestive system time to adjust.

- Drink plenty of water to help your body process the extra fiber and keep your bowels moving smoothly.

3 tricks to quick relief

Most hemorrhoids stop hurting on their own within a week or two, but, until then, they give you nothing but grief. Take some of the ache out with these simple, safe solutions.

Chill out. Kick back, put up your feet, and apply an ice pack or cold compress to hemorrhoids. Try this up to four times a day to soothe swelling.

Take a dip. Enjoy a warm soak for 15 minutes, three or four times a day. You don't need to run a full bath. Simply sit in a few inches of warm, not hot, water with your knees raised. Drugstores sell Sitz Baths, small soaking tubs that fit over an open toilet. Hold the bubbles and Epsom salts, though. These can irritate hemorrhoids.

Wipe on witch hazel. This herb is a natural astringent, helping shrink swollen tissue and ease throbbing pain. Look for moist cleansing cloths and pads made with witch hazel at your local drugstore.

Citrus-y supplement shuts down pain

Oranges and tangerines do more than load you up on vitamin C. They are also chock-full of lesser-known natural compounds called bioflavonoids. By strengthening the walls of your blood vessels, these compounds may treat blood vessel disorders such as hemorrhoids, nosebleeds, and bruising.

Experts tested a special, finely ground combination of hesperidin and diosmin, two citrus bioflavonoids, and found they worked especially well on hemorrhoids. In several strong studies, this combo-supplement cut the number and severity of hemorrhoid flare-ups, plus eased symptoms once an attack began. Look for a supplement made with 90 percent diosmin and 10 percent hesperidin. People in these trials tended to take it for at least two months.

Hiccups

Tried-and-true tricks to stop spasms

Let's face it – hiccups are funny. These silly noises make a normally dignified person sound like the town drunk in an old Western. The only things funnier than hiccups are some of the wacky folk remedies used to cure them. You can think of seven baldheaded men, roll down a grassy slope, put a penny in your navel, throw your arms in the air and spit three times, stand on one foot and hold your ears, hit yourself over the head with a newspaper, or hop up a flight of stairs with your feet together. But when you're done, you'll probably still have hiccups.

Of course, hiccups are less funny when they're happening to you. Then they can be downright annoying. Frustration sets in, and you wonder what's going on and why you can't stop it.

Here's what happens when hiccups strike. Somehow, the nerves that regulate breathing become irritated. They send a signal that causes your diaphragm to spasm and your glottis, the flap of skin at the top of your windpipe, to slam shut. This accounts for the distinctive hiccup sound.

Several things can trigger hiccups. Like the town drunk, you can drink too much. Alcohol may relax the nerves that normally keep hiccups in check. Overeating or eating too quickly, moving from a warm environment to a cold one or vice versa, and drinking carbonated beverages may also bring on hiccups. Rarely, hiccups – whose technical term is singultus – can be a symptom of a more serious problem, such as pneumonia, diabetes, heartburn, ulcers, tumors, multiple sclerosis, and stroke.

In extreme cases, you may need prescription drugs, acupuncture, or even surgery to get rid of a stubborn case of hiccups. Fortunately, hiccups are usually harmless – and humorous – nuisances that stop on their own after a few minutes. But if you want to speed them on their way, you can always try the following tried-and-true tips.

Simple ways to win relief

Hiccups wreak havoc with your normal breathing process. To make them go away, try these three simple breathing techniques.

Bag it. One popular – and effective – remedy involves breathing into a paper bag. This works by boosting the levels of carbon dioxide in your blood. As carbon dioxide levels go up, hiccups tend to clear up. Hold a brown paper bag around your nose and mouth and quickly breathe in and out about 15 times. Then take a deep breath, hold it for about 10 seconds, and breathe out. Repeat until the hiccups stop.

Hold it. Simply holding your breath can help. By interrupting the respiratory cycle, you nudge your nervous system back on track. Sneezing or coughing may also do the trick.

Triple it. Three's company when it comes to hiccup remedies. A cure called "supra-supra-maximal inspiration," described by doctors at the New York University School of Medicine, involves inhaling three times in a row. First, take a deep breath and hold it for 10 seconds. Without exhaling, breathe in again, pause, and then breathe in a third time. It's sort of a combination of breathing into a paper bag and holding your breath because you're increasing your carbon dioxide levels and interrupting the respiratory cycle.

No matter which breathing trick you choose, relief is only a few breaths away – and with hiccups out of the way, you can breathe a lot easier.

MythBuster: Can a "Boo!" banish hiccups?

You're hiccupping away, and suddenly your friend pops out from around a corner and yells "Boo!" Is your friend being helpful or just being a jerk? It depends on how you react. Being scared can stop hiccups. That's because when you gasp, as you would when you're startled, you interrupt the respiratory cycle. This jolt to the nervous system can reset the nerve impulse to your diaphragm and get your breathing back to normal. Next time you have hiccups, ask someone to scare you. Just relax and try not to anticipate the moment. Interestingly, while a well-timed "Boo!" can frighten away hiccups, shock and fear may also trigger them.

Drinking games douse hiccups

Hiccups got you down? Drink up. Several home remedies for hiccups involve drinking beverages. Here are some of the best ways to beat your hiccups.

- Drink from the far side of the glass. It's certainly awkward, but it may also be effective because it stimulates nerves in the back of the mouth, nose, and throat that aren't affected by normal drinking. This provides a shock to your nervous system – just the kind of spark you need to stop hiccups.
- Sip some ice water. The quick change in temperature in your esophagus may halt the hiccups.
- Sweeten the deal. Dissolve some sugar in a glass of water, and drink it. Simply swallowing a spoonful of sugar may also work.
- Drink a glass of water through a paper towel.
- Gargle to stimulate the nerves in your throat.

- Try sour power. Some people recommend gargling with cider vinegar. You can also just swallow a teaspoon of vinegar.

Other folk remedies include drinking pickle juice or eggshell tea, but that sounds worse than having the hiccups. You should also avoid drinking alcohol – too much of that can trigger hiccups in the first place.

Hands-on solutions to hiccup problem

When hiccups strike, sometimes it's best to take matters into your own hands. Check out these physical approaches to handling hiccups. While it may seem that these remedies – like hiccups –serve no purpose, the general idea is to stimulate or short-circuit the nerves that may control the hiccup impulse.

- With a spoon or cotton swab, gently lift the uvula, the V-shaped tissue hanging down at the back of your throat.
- Plug your ears for about 20 seconds.
- Massage your earlobes.
- Pull your tongue. Do this gently.
- Pinch your upper lip, just below your right nostril.
- Apply gentle pressure to your closed eyelids.

You may feel a bit silly trying some of these tricks, but you already sound silly with the hiccups. With nothing to lose – besides the hiccups – you may as well give these remedies a chance.

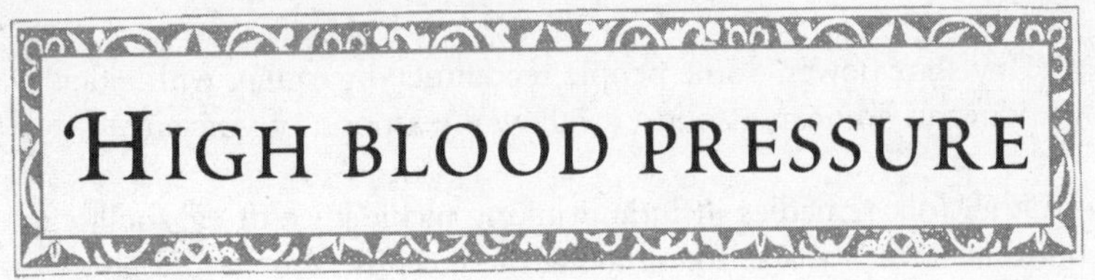

HIGH BLOOD PRESSURE

Super steps to head off trouble

Pressure can really take its toll. Just ask the student who failed the big test or the batter who struck out with the bases loaded. Your heart can also crack under too much pressure. When you have high blood pressure, or hypertension, your heart has to work harder than normal to pump blood through your circulatory system. This can damage both your heart and your arteries and boost your risk of heart attack, stroke, kidney disease, and blindness.

Know your numbers. Blood pressure, the force of your blood pushing against your artery walls, is measured in millimeters of mercury (mm) and includes two numbers. Systolic pressure, the top number, measures blood pressure when the heart contracts. Diastolic pressure, the bottom number, refers to blood pressure when the heart relaxes between contractions.

Because high blood pressure often has no outward symptoms, it's important to get your blood pressure checked by a doctor. Otherwise, you may not know you have high blood pressure until it's too late. Here's what your blood pressure reading means.

- Lower than 120/80(normal).
- 120-139/80-89 (prehypertension). Think of a blood pressure reading in this range as a warning sign. You are at risk for developing high blood pressure unless you start taking steps to get it under control.
- 140/90 or higher (high blood pressure).

Blood pressure increases with age. In fact, two-thirds of Americans over age 60 have high blood pressure. Blacks are also at high risk. Being overweight and inactive, smoking, drinking, stress, and a diet high in salt and fat can also contribute to this problem.

Take control. You can find plenty of unusual folk remedies for controlling high blood pressure. Putting mustard in your shoe, soaking your feet in hot water, or placing a violet-eyed grasshopper under your front steps are just a few examples. More than likely, your doctor will prescribe medication to lower your blood pressure. But in many cases, you can get your blood pressure under control with a few simple lifestyle changes.

- Lose weight if you're overweight.
- Eat a healthy diet.
- Cut back on salt.
- Exercise regularly.
- Reduce stress.
- Quit smoking.
- Drink alcohol in moderation (if at all). This means no more than two drinks a day for a man and one for a woman.

DASH lowers BP in a flash

What you put on your plate can make the difference between high blood pressure and healthy blood pressure. For the best nutritional advice, check out the Dietary Approaches to Stop Hypertension (DASH) eating plan. Developed by the National Heart, Lung, and Blood Institute, DASH features the following key recommendations.

- Cut down on saturated fat, total fat, and cholesterol.
- Eat more fruits and vegetables.
- Make room for fat-free or low-fat milk and milk products.

Common fruit juice poses big risk

Normally, grapefruit juice is a healthy beverage – but if you're taking calcium channel blockers to control your high blood pressure, it can be dangerous. That's because substances in grapefruit juice called furanocoumarins interact with the medication, causing your body to absorb too much of it. This can lead to a dangerous drop in blood pressure or an alarmingly rapid heartbeat. Grapefruit juice also interacts with several other drugs, including statins and antidepressants. Ask your doctor if it's safe to drink grapefruit juice with your medication. Or just play it safe and choose orange juice instead.

- Include whole grain products, fish, poultry, and nuts.
- Reduce red meat, sweets, added sugars, and sugary drinks.
- Get plenty of potassium, magnesium, calcium, fiber, and protein.

Studies show the DASH plan works as well as commonly prescribed blood pressure drugs – and it works fast. Within two weeks, you can lower your blood pressure. The plan becomes even more effective if you also limit your salt intake.

Enjoy extra benefits. As a bonus, DASH does more than just lower blood pressure. It also lowers LDL, or bad cholesterol, further reducing your risk of heart disease. Flush arteries clean of plaque and fatty buildup with this highly effective, all-natural, and completely safe treatment. Rich in disease-fighting phytochemicals, thanks to all the fruits and vegetables, DASH may even protect against cancer.

Cut back on carbs. DASH works just fine as it is, but with a few tweaks, it may work even better. One study found that two reduced-carbohydrate versions of DASH outperformed the original DASH plan. One plan substituted 10 percent of DASH's carbohydrate calories with protein from plant sources, chicken, and egg whites, while the other swapped the carbs for healthy unsaturated fats, like olive or canola oils.

Get moving. Whether you stick to the original DASH plan or try one of the modified versions, your best bet is to combine the plan with lifestyle changes, like weight loss and exercise. Aim for at least 30 minutes of moderate exercise, like walking, jogging, swimming, or cycling, a day.

You don't even have to set aside one block of time for your workout. Three or four brisk 10-minute walks may work even better than one longer stroll. The important thing is to increase your physical activity – even if it's just everyday tasks, like cleaning your house, washing dishes, doing yard work, washing your car, or going up and down the stairs. Every little bit of activity helps.

Eat to beat high blood pressure

You don't have to reach into your medicine cabinet to control your blood pressure. Go to your garden (or grocery) for a truly effective way to relieve high blood pressure. Garlic is the key – it adds flavor to your food while subtracting millimeters of mercury from your blood pressure reading. Thanks to garlic's sulfur compounds and flavonoids, this fragrant herb is one folk remedy that really works. In addition to garlic, the following foods may help get your blood pressure down to a healthy level.

- **Bananas.** Eating just two bananas a day can drop your blood pressure by 10 percent. That's because bananas are good sources of potassium, which helps regulate blood pressure.

- **Celery.** This crunchy vegetable, used in traditional Chinese medicine, contains compounds called pthalides that relax blood vessels and reduce stress hormones.

- **Chocolate.** You don't want to eat too much of this sweet treat, but a little bit of flavonoid-rich dark chocolate may help lower blood pressure.

- **Flaxseeds.** These little nutritional powerhouses are rich in omega-3 fatty acids, the same polyunsaturated fats that help fish tame high blood pressure.

- **Potatoes.** Scientists recently discovered that potatoes contain chemicals called kukoamines that lower blood pressure. For best results, boil rather than fry your taters.

- **Tomatoes.** A small study found that a tomato extract supplement lowered blood pressure. Rich in lycopene, tomatoes and tomato products may provide the same benefits.

Terrific tips to sidestep salt

Salt looks harmless enough, but don't let its innocent appearance fool you. Higher salt intake means higher blood pressure. That's because salt causes your body to retain water, increasing the amount of blood in your arteries. It also causes small arteries to constrict, making it harder for blood to get through.

Experts recommend you get no more than 2,300 milligrams (mg) of sodium – roughly equal to one teaspoon of salt – a day. If you have high blood pressure, you should cut that down to 1,500 mg or less. Right now, the average American consumes more than 4,000 mg of sodium daily. Just laying off the saltshaker won't solve the problem. Most sodium hides in prepared foods, so it's hard to know how much salt you're getting. To combat this problem, the American Medical Association (AMA) has urged restaurants and manufacturers to reduce their sodium by a minimum of 50 percent in the next decade. Until then, you can take the following steps.

Spice things up. You don't need salt to season your food. Avoid high blood pressure and add delicious flavor to your meals with these spices. As a bonus, they're also rich in antioxidants. Try ground cloves, ground cinnamon, and oregano for the most antioxidant punch. Other flavorful alternatives to salt include basil, bay leaf, chili powder, cumin, curry powder, dry mustard, garlic powder, ginger, onion powder, paprika, parsley, black or red pepper, poultry seasoning, thyme, and turmeric.

MythBuster: Can doctors cause high BP?

You rely on your doctor to check your blood pressure – but he could be part of the problem. Up to 35 percent of people with high blood pressure have a condition called "white coat hypertension." This means your blood pressure is high when checked by a doctor or in a medical environment, but normal otherwise. Fortunately, you can buy a home monitor and check your blood pressure yourself. This will give you a more accurate measurement of your usual blood pressure. Having your blood pressure checked by a nurse rather than a doctor may also help.

Read labels. Pay attention to the sodium content of the foods you buy. Look for items marked "no salt added," "low sodium," or "reduced sodium."

Do it yourself. Your best bet is to cut back on restaurant meals and processed foods, like cold cuts, canned vegetables, canned soups, frozen dinners, cheeses, salad dressings, snack foods, and fast foods. When you prepare your own meals from scratch, it's harder for salt to sneak up on you.

5 delicious drinks drop BP

Raise your glass and lower your blood pressure. Simply sipping the following beverages may help.

Water. Lowering high blood pressure levels can be as easy as drinking more water. Choosing this natural beverage instead of sugary drinks has a positive impact on your whole body. Try mineral water that is rich in magnesium. Studies show this mineral, along with potassium and calcium, helps regulate blood pressure.

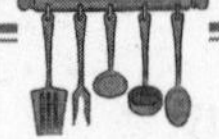

Green tea can fight heart disease, cancer, even allergies. Follow these brewing tips to make the most of this healthy beverage. First, make sure to use fresh, good-quality water. The right proportion is also important. Use 8 ounces of water for every heaping teaspoon of green tea. Two minutes is enough time for the tea to brew. You'll end up with bitter tea if you let it brew too long or if your water is too hot. For best results, use a Japanese teapot specially designed for green tea.

Tea. Brew yourself a longer life with the world's second favorite beverage. You already know that No. 1 – water – is good for you, too. An Australian study found that each daily cup of tea dropped systolic blood pressure by 2 points and diastolic pressure by 1 point. Green tea also may reduce the risk of coronary artery disease and heart attack.

Fermented milk. If you want something more unusual, try this traditional Scandinavian drink that lowered blood pressure in a Finnish study.

Low-fat milk. Your milk doesn't have to be fermented to knock your blood pressure down a few points. Just make sure it's low in fat. Studies show low-fat dairy products reduce your risk of developing high blood pressure.

Grape juice. A Korean study found that Concord grape juice, which is rich in polyphenols, lowers blood pressure.

On the other hand, some beverages do more harm than good. For instance, beer and wine both raise blood pressure. Caffeinated drinks also pose a problem. Coffee boosts blood pressure in the short term, but its long-term effects on blood pressure remain unclear. However, colas – even diet colas – may increase your risk of developing high blood pressure. Beware of energy drinks, which contain up to four times the caffeine of a regular soda.

High cholesterol

Proven ways to de-clutter your arteries

Your attic or basement may be overflowing with collections, family heirlooms, or just old things you can't bear to throw away. When the clutter starts creeping into your living area, it can become a nuisance – and even a fire hazard. Think of your cholesterol like clutter. What begins with just the essentials can quickly escalate into a major problem.

Keep it down. Your body needs cholesterol, a soft, waxy substance essential for building cell walls and making hormones. But you can get too much of a good thing. When you take in too much cholesterol, it builds up on your artery walls and causes blockages that lead to heart attack or stroke.

Not all cholesterol is the same. Just as your clutter can be divided into categories – photographs, furniture, knick knacks – your cholesterol also has distinct varieties.

- LDL. Low-density lipoprotein is considered "bad" because it carries cholesterol to your artery walls where it can do damage.
- HDL. High-density lipoprotein, or good cholesterol, whisks cholesterol to your liver, where it is eliminated.
- Triglycerides. These lipids, or fats, may lead to blood clots and inflammation. They may also lower HDL levels.

Check it out. Like high blood pressure, high cholesterol can sneak up on you because it has no outer symptoms. Unless you get your cholesterol levels measured by a doctor, you may not know you have a problem until it's too late. A simple blood test does the trick. Cholesterol and triglycerides are measured in milligrams per deciliter of blood, or mg/dL. Your numbers to strive for vary depending on your level of risk for heart disease. The higher your risk, the lower you want your LDL. Your doctor will help you determine your target levels. Here are some general goals to keep in mind.

- Total cholesterol – less than 200 mg/dL is desirable. Between 200 and 239 is borderline, and over 240 is high.
- LDL – below 100 mg/dL is ideal. If you're at very high risk, you should aim even lower – 70 mg/dL. Anything over 160 is high, while levels above 190 are very high and require medication.
- HDL – above 40 mg/dL is desirable, while levels above 60 mg/dL are optimal.
- Triglycerides – below 150 mg/dL is normal, from 150 to 199 is borderline high, and from 200-499 is high. Over 500 is very high.

Take control. Your cholesterol tends to increase with age. Family history also plays a role. While you can't change your age or your genetics, you can take steps to battle other risk factors, including obesity, inactivity, and an unhealthy diet. Eating right, exercising regularly, losing weight, and quitting smoking go a long way toward lowering your cholesterol. Your doctor may also prescribe drugs – like statins – to keep your cholesterol under control. Even if you need medication, that doesn't mean you should rely on drugs alone. Stick to a healthy lifestyle and your drugs will work even better.

Healthy diet hammers high cholesterol

Think you can beat high cholesterol without changing your diet? Fat chance. To lower your cholesterol, you need to eat right – and that means focusing on fats. Here are the main types of fats and how much you should eat of each.

- **Saturated fat.** Nothing raises your cholesterol more than saturated fat. Found in meat and whole milk dairy products, saturated fat raises bad LDL cholesterol and increases your risk

Beware of sneaky labels

Now that manufacturers must list trans fats on their product labels, you'd think it would be easier to avoid these harmful fats, which raise bad LDL cholesterol and lower good HDL cholesterol. But that's not the case. In fact, products can boast "0 grams trans fat" as long as they have less than .5 grams per serving. So you may be eating trans fats without even knowing it. Worse yet, products loaded with saturated fat can claim, truthfully, that they contain "0 grams trans fat." But that doesn't make them healthy foods. Pay close attention to food labels and ingredient lists to avoid being misled.

of heart disease. Less than 7 percent of your daily calories should come from saturated fat.

- **Monounsaturated fat.** Found in olive oil and canola oil, this healthy fat may lower LDL cholesterol while boosting protective HDL cholesterol. It should make up about 10-15 percent of your calories.
- **Polyunsaturated fat.** Vegetable oils, nuts, and fish contain polyunsaturated fat, which helps lower cholesterol. About 10 percent of your calories should come from polyunsaturated fats.
- **Trans fats.** These harmful fats, formed when manufacturers add hydrogen to unsaturated fat to make it more solid, raise LDL and may lower HDL. You can find trans fats in stick margarine, baked goods, and French fries. Limit trans fats as much as possible.

All fats pack 9 calories per gram, so you should keep your total fat intake to about 30 percent of your daily calories. While fats have the biggest impact on your cholesterol levels, you also want to limit the cholesterol you get from foods – like egg yolks, liver, shrimp, and whole-milk dairy products – to 200 milligrams a day.

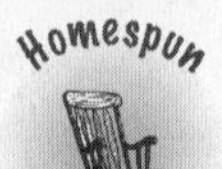

Old remedy may still work

One of the staples of traditional European medicine – the artichoke – may help lower your cholesterol in the present day. Artichoke leaves contain a compound called cynarin that blocks cholesterol synthesis. In fact, synthetic cynarin was used to treat high cholesterol until the 1980s. Some recent studies show artichoke leaf extract – and even frozen artichoke juice – lower cholesterol. You can try the dried herb or just eat some artichokes. Just make sure not to counteract their health benefits by dipping the leaves in a rich, buttery sauce. Try a yogurt-based dip instead.

On the other hand, you want to make room for more soluble fiber and plant sterols and stanols, which block the absorption of cholesterol as it moves through your digestive tract. Aim for 10 to 25 daily grams of soluble fiber, which you'll find in oats, barley, beans, and fruits and vegetables. Look for margarines or other foods, like orange juice, that have been fortified with plant sterols or stanols. Just 2 grams a day helps lower cholesterol.

Changing your diet can lead to a healthy change in your cholesterol levels. In fact, Canadian researchers found that a diet high in plant sterols, almonds, soy protein, and soluble fiber from oats, barley, psyllium, okra, and eggplant, worked about as well as the cholesterol-lowering drug lovastatin.

Pros and cons of OTC heart helpers

Not every cure for high cholesterol comes with a prescription. Several herbs and supplements claim to lower cholesterol. Here's a look at some of them, along with those you should watch out for.

Berberine. Here's some good heart news. Scientists now say this traditional Chinese herb, formerly used to fight diarrhea, may help lower cholesterol. In a Chinese study, three months of berberine lowered total cholesterol by 29 percent, triglycerides by 35 percent, and LDL cholesterol by 25 percent. Here's more good news – it's cheap. For about 70 cents a day, berberine could be a low-cost option in the fight against high cholesterol.

Cholest-Off. This blend of plant sterols and stanols helps block the absorption of cholesterol in your bloodstream. Unlike margarines or other foods fortified with sterols or stanols, this supplement offers cholesterol-lowering benefits without any additional calories.

Coenzyme Q10. If you take statins, this natural supplement may help with side effects like muscle pain or damage. People who experience side effects from statins often have low levels of this important enzyme in their blood.

Psyllium. Take some of this soluble fiber supplement, and you may be able to cut down on your dosage of prescription drugs. One study found that 10 milligrams of the cholesterol-lowering drug simvastatin plus 15 grams of psyllium worked just as well as 20 mg of the drug alone.

Red yeast rice. This Chinese supplement may contain natural lovastatin, making it an effective way to lower LDL and triglycerides. But legal issues have taken it off the market in the United States. If you do find it, you can't be sure you're getting enough of the active ingredient because the lovastatin levels are no longer standardized.

Niacin. One of the more effective remedies for high cholesterol, niacin significantly raises HDL and lowers LDL and triglycerides. But this vitamin comes with the risk of serious side effects and should not be taken without a doctor's supervision.

Policosanol. You may have heard some glowing reports about this supplement made from sugarcane. But a recent German study found policosanol worked no better than a placebo, or dummy pill, in lowering cholesterol. Previous supportive studies were funded by the Cuban marketer of the supplement.

Guggul. Stay away from this herbal supplement, especially if you take prescription drugs. Guggulsterone, the active ingredient in guggul, reduces the effectiveness of more than half of all prescription drugs, including statins. Besides, it may not even work. While some studies show guggul lowers cholesterol, a recent University of Pennsylvania study found that it actually raised LDL levels if taken at high doses.

Supermarket savvy to control cholesterol

You already know a healthy diet helps lower your cholesterol. But when you put the following foods and beverages on your menu, you may get an extra boost in your battle against high cholesterol.

Barley. Like oats, barley is a good source of the soluble fiber beta-glucan, which helps lower cholesterol. In one study, people who ate 3 grams or 6 grams of beta-glucan each day through foods like pancakes and muffins made with barley significantly lowered their LDL and total cholesterol. Just beware of adding too much too quickly. You may experience bloating and gas.

Broccoli sprouts. Just one week of eating broccoli sprouts may lower your total and LDL cholesterol while boosting your HDL.

Fish. Rich in omega-3 fatty acids, fish lowers triglycerides and may raise good HDL cholesterol. However, it may also raise your LDL. When you pair fish with garlic, you get the best of both worlds. If you're worried about mercury poisoning from fish, you can also get similar benefits from flax, another source of omega-3.

Nuts. Grab a handful of almonds, walnuts, pecans, or pistachios for a healthy snack that crunches cholesterol. Even peanuts – technically legumes and not nuts – can help. Keep in mind that nuts, while healthy, are also high in fat. So don't go nuts with nuts.

Black tea. Enjoy afternoon tea, and bid high cholesterol goodnight. Five cups of flavonoid-rich black tea per day can significantly reduce total and LDL cholesterol.

MythBuster: Should you avoid eggs?

You may consider eggs a dietary no-no, along with fatty or fried foods. In fact, research shows an egg a day does not increase heart disease risk in healthy people. Egg yolks have a lot of cholesterol, but the cholesterol you get from food only affects your blood cholesterol slightly. Saturated fat does much more damage. Eggs also provide heart-healthy nutrients like protein, vitamins B12 and D, riboflavin, and folate. Still, if you have trouble controlling your cholesterol, you may want to choose egg whites – which have no cholesterol – instead.

Tomato juice. It only takes two daily cups of tomato juice to lower cholesterol. That's enough to increase LDL's resistance to oxidation by about 42 percent. After oxidation, LDL becomes more dangerous, so preventing oxidation helps protect your heart. The lycopene in tomato juice does the trick.

Cranberry juice. Like tomato juice, cranberry juice also inhibits LDL oxidation. It may also boost HDL levels.

Small changes make a big difference

If you think you have no time for breakfast, think again. Skipping breakfast can lead to higher cholesterol and weight gain. Start each day off right with a healthy breakfast like whole-grain cereal, oatmeal, yogurt, or fruit, and help put an end to high cholesterol. Eating breakfast is just one easy step you can take. Here are some other simple, natural remedies that can lower your cholesterol, clean your arteries, and reduce your blood pressure – for good.

Exercise regularly. You may have trouble finding time to exercise, but surely you have three minutes to spare. A recent study found that

10 three-minute exercise sessions worked as well as one 30-minute session to lower triglycerides. Physical activity also boosts HDL and helps keep your weight under control, which reduces LDL. Even if you're naturally thin, you should exercise. Sedentary thin people have high cholesterol, just like inactive overweight people. Aim for at least 30 minutes of moderate exercise a day.

Marinating your meat will help keep it from forming unhealthy cholesterol oxidation products during cooking, which can lead to heart disease and cancer. According to one study, an effective marinade mixes 10 percent soy sauce, 1 percent sugar, and 89 percent water. You can convert that to 10 tablespoons (5 ounces) soy sauce, 1 tablespoon sugar, and 5½ cups of water.

Lose weight. When you are overweight, you are more likely to have high triglycerides and LDL and low HDL. You also boost your risk of high blood pressure, diabetes, heart disease, and other serious health problems. To get down to a healthy weight, you need to burn more calories than you take in. The best way to do that is a combination of a healthy diet and exercise.

Quit smoking. Cigarette smoking raises your LDL cholesterol and lowers your HDL cholesterol. It also contributes to blood clots and hardening of the arteries. Even second-hand smoke can harm you. Break the habit as soon as possible.

Reduce stress. You know stress can send your blood pressure skyrocketing – but it may also raise your cholesterol. Find ways to reduce or cope with stress. Listening to music, exercising, and relaxation techniques can help.

Get religion. A University of Pittsburgh Medical Center study found that attending weekly religious services helps people live longer. In fact, religious attendance is almost as helpful in adding years to your life as regular exercise and statins.

Insomnia

Easy remedies to bring on sleep

"Oh sleep! it is a gentle thing, Beloved from pole to pole," wrote the English poet Samuel Taylor Coleridge. If you've ever had trouble drifting off to the land of Nod, you know what it's like to lie in bed unable to get your 40 winks, wishing for some "beloved" sleep.

Insomnia, from the Latin words meaning "no sleep," can be a short-term problem for some people, but it's a chronic complaint for others. About 60 million Americans every year say they have trouble sleeping. You may be unable to fall asleep or stay asleep because of physical problems like illness or surgery, stress over a job or family concern, or even bothersome bedroom conditions when you travel. Women often have trouble sleeping when their hormone levels rise and fall. If your insomnia is caused by a health problem that makes you uncomfortable and robs you of sleep, it's called secondary insomnia. But if your sleeplessness is not due to illness, it's primary insomnia.

You may think you can learn to get by on less sleep, but don't fool yourself. Not getting the seven or eight hours most adults need simply runs up a "sleep debt," which you have to pay back some time. If you don't get enough sleep, you'll probably feel tired and grumpy the next day and have trouble concentrating and remembering things. That's annoying, but it can also be dangerous. Studies show driving drowsy is as dangerous as driving drunk, with sleepy drivers causing around 200,000 accidents each year. Plus, if you don't get your Z's on a regular basis you're more likely to be overweight, and you're at risk for diabetes and depression.

You've probably heard loads of advice on getting to sleep, since most people have a favorite trick – from counting sheep to saying the Lord's Prayer backwards to eating a raw onion before bed. Drugs are available, but many have side effects, and none can cure chronic insomnia. Changing the way you live is a simpler and more effective

Sleepy-time secrets

Poor habits or a sloppy bedtime routine can cause trouble sleeping. Try these 10 easy tips for sound and restful sleep every night.

- Stick to a regular sleep schedule, or regular time for going to bed and getting up, even on the weekends.
- Don't nap in the late afternoon or evening.
- Keep your bedroom cool and dark.
- Don't live in bed. Use it only for sleeping and sex.
- Avoid too much caffeine, especially in the evenings.
- Don't smoke. Nicotine can keep you awake.
- Eat a light snack near bedtime, but don't fill up with a heavy meal too late in the day.
- Check your medicine. Some drugs, like antidepressants and beta blockers, can cause you to stay awake.
- Spend about 30 minutes in the sun during the day to reset your body's clock.
- Don't watch the clock if you can't sleep. After 15 or 20 minutes of lying awake, get up and do something different until you feel sleepy.

way to treat your problem. Check out these cheap and natural remedies that will soon have you snoozing like Rip Van Winkle.

Relaxation puts your mind at rest

Worrying about problems and planning for the next day can keep you awake at night – even if you've followed all the rules for good sleep habits. William Shakespeare was right when he said, "where care lodges, sleep will never lie." What can you do to relax your mind and stop the worrying?

Researchers tested various behavioral methods, or ways of changing how you think about sleep, and pitted them against taking sleeping pills. They looked at progressive muscle relaxation, biofeedback, cognitive behavioral therapy (CBT), and other techniques.

Taking drugs to bring on sleep works, but it's not as fast as behavioral changes, and people can come to rely on sleeping pills. Also, scientists say changing people's thoughts can actually cure insomnia in the long run, unlike drugs. In one study, researchers found CBT – talk therapy with a counselor – worked better than sleeping pills for people with chronic insomnia.

You can seek help from a professional, or you can try to improve your own thought patterns. Pay attention to your beliefs about sleep and sleeplessness. Try to change negative thoughts like "I'll never survive tomorrow if I don't get to sleep soon," to positive ideas like "I'll bet I'm actually getting more rest than I think." Don't get preoccupied by the idea of insomnia, and don't watch the minutes tick by as you lie awake.

Finally, if your thoughts are still racing ahead to tomorrow's problems, get up and write down the trouble that's keeping you awake. Sometimes putting it on paper can put your mind at rest. Your body will soon follow.

MythBuster: Do older people need less sleep?

It would be nice to get by on less sleep, but that's not a benefit of going gray. Adults of all ages need the same seven or eight hours of sleep nightly. Unfortunately, as you age, you spend less time in deep sleep, so you may awaken more easily. Sleep cycles can also shift, so you fall asleep and wake up earlier than when you were young. Add that to the fact that seniors often have more health problems, take drugs that disrupt sleep, and awaken to urinate at night, and it's no wonder you may no longer sleep like a baby.

Snooze news: time to 'retire' old tricks

Everyone has a favorite method of getting to sleep, but some ideas are as useless as the old wives' tales of putting a horseshoe under your bed or a pair of scissors beneath your pillow. You may have even tried some of these old standards and been disappointed with the results. Here's why.

Use alcohol sparingly. Some people think a drink with alcohol will help them sleep, but alcohol disrupts your sleep cycle. Although it may help you fall asleep more easily, you'll skip the deeper, more restful stages and stay in light sleep, so you're more likely to be disturbed before the night is over.

Save warm milk for the baby. The idea behind this remedy is that milk's tryptophan, a building block of protein, helps make natural melatonin to put you to sleep. It's great in theory, but an 8-ounce glass of milk doesn't have enough tryptophan to work. Instead, try a 3-ounce snack of turkey, which has seven times as much tryptophan.

Take an early bath. A hot bath at bedtime can make you more alert – just what you don't want at that time of day. If you find a hot bath soothing, take it an hour and a half to two hours before bed.

Daytime activity promotes nighttime rest

Remember the good old days of childhood, when you fell asleep as soon as your head hit the pillow? That was probably after a day of running, playing ball, or riding your bicycle. By evening you were drained and ready for rest. The same can be true for adults of all ages – exercise can help you get to sleep.

Scientists tested the importance of exercise along with socializing on a group of older adults. They developed a program of daily fitness activities, including stretching, walking, dancing, and doing calisthenics as a group. The 90-minute program also included some just-for-fun pursuits like playing cards or board games to encourage chatting and interaction.

After two weeks, most people in the study reported they slept better and were in brighter moods than before the program. They also scored higher on mental tests. Another study found exercise could work as well as sleeping pills to help you sleep.

Finish your vigorous exercise early in the day rather than just before bedtime. Too much physical activity in the evening can lower your body's level of melatonin, a natural hormone that gets you ready for sleep. Instead, gentle stretching exercises in the evening can help relax you for bed.

Melatonin restores rhythm of sleep

Back in the days of horse-drawn wagons and candlelight, people got up with the sun and went to sleep when evening fell. Now electricity gives light at any time – yet most people still sleep at night and get up near dawn. How does your body know what time it is?

Daylight and certain natural chemicals control your body's daily biological clock, or circadian rhythm. The hormone melatonin, made in the brain, lets your body know it's getting dark outside and it's time for you to sleep. But if you change your body's clock by working the night shift or traveling across time zones, your melatonin

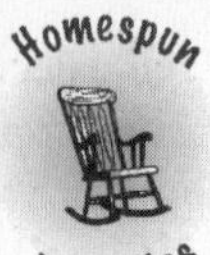

Flowery brew brings on sweet dreams

Chamomile tea is an old favorite remedy for sleeplessness that just may work for you. The herb it's made from contains certain natural chemicals, or flavenoids, that act on your brain just like a sleeping pill. As an added bonus, this soothing bedtime drink can also calm an upset stomach and treat diarrhea and gas. But if you're allergic to plants in the ragweed family, you may want to avoid chamomile. And don't drink chamomile tea if you take sleeping pills or other drugs that affect your nervous system.

level can be thrown off. As people get older they also tend to produce less melatonin, making sleep harder to grasp.

You can buy melatonin in the form of pills or liquid, but experts disagree on how much to take. Most common pills are 3 to 5 milligrams (mg), a fairly large dose that is not helpful for typical insomnia. "After a few days it stops working," says Professor Richard Wurtman, a researcher at Massachusetts Institute of Technology who studies brain chemicals and sleep. His research shows this dose is too high and may actually keep you awake longer. Instead, try a smaller dose of about 0.3 mg (300 mcg) melatonin.

Melatonin is most helpful if your sleep trouble is due to the following conditions:

- jet lag
- blindness, which can block your body's natural light cues
- delayed sleep syndrome, or trouble falling asleep until late at night
- old age

Don't take melatonin if you have liver or kidney problems or you are depressed.

Valerian: a ticket to the land of Nod

Eating a spoonful of peanut butter, drinking peppermint or snake-root tea, and chewing poppy flowers were once recommended as evening snacks to bring on sleep. Valerian root is another time-tested herbal tonic, and science proves it works.

This herb contains many compounds, and researchers don't know which ones help you sleep. One theory is that valeric acid, a main ingredient, changes the levels of enzymes in your brain to make you calm and ready for rest. No matter how valerian works, studies show it's as effective as some common sleeping pills like oxazepam and triazolam. Even better, the herb doesn't cause the same side effects that sleeping pills can have, like morning grogginess or difficulty thinking clearly.

Valerian

You can brew a cup of valerian tea for a mild effect or take the herb in the form of capsules. A commonly researched dosage is 600 milligrams about an hour before bedtime. Just be aware that you may have to take the herb for several weeks before you feel its effect.

As with all herbal supplements, stick to a reputable brand. The Food and Drug Administration does not regulate herbal supplements, so some don't actually contain the amount listed on the label, and they may be contaminated. Valerian can cause vivid dreams, and you shouldn't use it if you drink alcohol regularly or take sleeping pills.

IRRITABLE BOWEL SYNDROME

Soothing solutions for IBS woes

Mark Twain said, "Part of the secret of success in life is to eat what you like and let the food fight it out inside." He also said, "To eat is human, to digest, divine." Sounds like a man who had experience with digestive problems.

Ever wonder why you sometimes have belly pain, gas, bloating, and either diarrhea or constipation – and you haven't eaten anything strange? Does your diarrhea strike so suddenly you have to run to the bathroom? Are these troubles even worse when something goes wrong in your life? You may suffer from irritable bowel syndrome (IBS), a collection of problems also referred to as spastic colon.

Don't confuse IBS with the more serious digestive problem, inflammatory bowel disease (IBD). People with IBS don't seem to have anything wrong with the structure of their digestive systems, but for some reason their colons don't work right. They are oversensitive to certain triggers, like some foods and emotional events. IBS can cause mostly diarrhea, mostly constipation, or even a combination of the two problems. One in five Americans suffer from IBS, the majority of them women. It's just a nuisance for some, but for the more unfortunate, life revolves around trips to the bathroom.

Your doctor may ask if you have bowel movements that are more or less frequent than usual, if your stool is watery or hard, and if the pain lessens after a bowel movement. If you've had unexplained belly pain and these symptoms for 12 weeks out of the past 12 months, you might be due for an IBS diagnosis.

Drugs and laxatives may work if you have serious IBS problems, but most doctors prefer you try natural relief first, by changing the way you live. These simple tips can help.

- Eat slowly so you don't swallow too much air.
- Drink six to eight glasses of water every day.
- Exercise to keep your digestive system moving and regular.
- Nix the caffeine, tobacco, alcohol, and chewing gum.
- Find ways to relax and cut back on emotional stress, which can disturb your colon.
- Keep track of what you eat, how you feel, and what IBS symptoms you have so you can identify your personal problem foods.

Food and fiber: the good, bad, and ugly

What you eat affects your health, especially when it comes to IBS. Careful food choices can be especially helpful if diarrhea is a major problem for you. Doctors prefer treating IBS this way because more than half of people get relief.

Try an elimination diet to determine which foods cause you the most trouble. Start by eating only bland, simple foods for a while,

Steer clear of certain sweeteners

Keep tabs on the sugars in your diet. Sorbitol, an artificial sweetener used in sugar-free chewing gum and diet candy, can make IBS symptoms worse. Sorbitol is not absorbed well in the small intestine, leaving it to cause trouble in your colon. If you notice worse bloating, gas, cramps, and diarrhea after you eat a lot of sorbitol, you may be oversensitive. Fructose, a natural sugar that gives fruit its sweetness, can cause similar problems for some people.

then gradually add other foods, and keep track of changes in your body. Keep a journal of foods that bring on symptoms, and show it to your doctor.

Foods that tend to make IBS symptoms worse include:

- drinks and food with caffeine, like coffee and chocolate.
- dairy products with lactose, including milk and ice cream.
- gassy vegetables such as broccoli and beans.
- fatty foods like french fries or cheese.

Adding fiber to your diet can help both constipation and diarrhea. Soluble fiber, found in psyllium husks, guar gum, fruit pectin, and oatmeal, soaks up water to create a gooey gel. This kind of fiber slows down food as it moves through your intestines.

Wheat

Insoluble fiber, from wheat bran and the peel of fruits, adds bulk to stool and helps it move through your gut more quickly. Soluble fiber seems to be the most helpful for IBS. But increase the fiber in your diet gradually to avoid causing even more gas and bloating. Finally, be sure to balance the extra fiber with enough water to keep things moving smoothly.

Probiotics provide bacterial balance

Some doctors think IBS is related to an imbalance of bacteria, or microflora, in your intestines. That's right – your innards need a healthy balance of "good" germs to function well and keep the disease-causing critters from taking over. Eating the wrong foods, taking antibiotics, or being under stress can upset the balance. Probiotics, certain strains of friendly bacteria added to foods or in pills, can put the microflora back in balance.

Doctors researching IBS believe too many of the wrong bacteria take over in the digestive system, even moving from the colon to the small intestine, where they don't belong. That overgrowth can cause the gas, bloating, diarrhea, and constipation of IBS. Several studies have shown that certain probiotics can cut back on these annoying IBS symptoms. The probiotics that seem most helpful for IBS include certain strains of *Lactobacillus* and some kinds of *Bifidobacteria*. *Lactobacillus* keeps disease-causing bacteria from attaching to the wall of the intestines. *Bifidobacteria* works by changing carbohydrates in the food you eat into acids that keep harmful bacteria from reproducing. When the bad bacteria can't grow, they don't put out harmful toxins into your gut.

You can get the right probiotics in the form of supplements, or you can eat yogurt that proclaims "live active yogurt cultures" on the label. Look for brands like Stonyfield Farm and Dannon Activia yogurt or DanActive yogurt drink. A recent study found the probiotic yogurt has more friendly bugs in each serving than the supplements, plus you get the added bonus of calcium and other nutrients.

Calm your nerves and your colon

Certain foods and stressful events in your life can trigger IBS symptoms. Both can cause an oversensitive colon to have spasms. This brain–belly connection is related to the enteric nervous system (ENS), a network of nerve cells controlling your stomach, intestines, and other digestive organs.

Fennel battles digestive upset

They taste a bit like licorice, and they're long known to banish many digestive woes. Fennel seeds may help with the diarrhea, constipation, gas, and cramps of IBS. The essential oils from fennel seeds keep the digestive system's involuntary muscles from having spasms. That helps your colon move smoothly and comfortably. Fennel is also a mild remedy for the excess gas that causes bloating. You can chew whole fennel seeds, like those offered in Indian restaurants, or brew a cup of fennel tea.

Neurotransmitters like serotonin, which exist in your gut as well as your brain, have been linked to IBS. When problems in your life affect your serotonin levels, they impact both your brain and your ENS. That's why some people suffer from diarrhea, constipation, or stomach pains when life gets too exciting.

You can deal with these stresses in many ways. Some people are helped by biofeedback, relaxation therapy, or talking to a counselor. You may be able to keep a lid on your stress level on your own by trying these simple ideas.

Get some exercise. Besides helping your digestive system work smoothly, aerobic exercise like walking or swimming puts more endorphins into your blood. These brain chemicals put you in a better mood and lighten your mental weight.

Keep a "stress diary." Each day, write down things that bother you as well as difficult events you encounter, along with your emotions at the time. Also include information about your IBS symptoms, including pain, gas, diarrhea, and constipation. When you see a link, you'll know what kinds of trouble to avoid.

MythBuster: Is it all in your head?

Some people can't sleep when they get upset, while others have digestive troubles. That means their symptoms are all in their heads, right? Not so fast. The colon muscles of someone with IBS are oversensitive, so stress or certain food makes the muscles contract too much. Even worse, people with severe IBS sometimes get depressed or worried about their symptoms, making for a vicious cycle. But IBS is a problem with the way the digestive system functions – it's not a psychological problem or personality disorder. Therapy or relaxation may help, but trigger foods will still bring on trouble.

Breathe easy. With one hand on your stomach, take a slow deep breath in while you count to four. Then breathe out while you count backwards to one.

Do what you like. Have you been neglecting your gardening, needlework, favorite novel, or woodworking tools? Devote some time to the hobby you enjoy most, and your stress may go out the window – taking IBS with it.

Get your beauty rest. People who don't treat themselves to enough sleep each night have more health problems, including worse IBS symptoms the next day.

Melatonin makes for a happy colon

Some people take melatonin to help them sleep, and it may also help IBS symptoms. Melatonin is made naturally in your brain and digestive system, and it keeps your biological clock ticking to let you sleep at night. Doctors aren't sure why melatonin helps IBS, but they think it blocks another brain chemical, serotonin, from working in the intestines.

Two recent studies found people with IBS who took 3 milligrams (mg) of melatonin every evening had relief. In one study, people who took the supplement for eight weeks had less abdominal pain and bloating, but the melatonin didn't change their problems with constipation or diarrhea. In the second study, people who took melatonin every evening had less pain and bloating, plus they had better moods and felt more in control of their lives. Both studies were small, so researchers want to test melatonin again to see how it affects other people.

With some brands of melatonin costing about six cents a day for 3-mg doses, it may be a simple and cheap way to get control over your IBS. But talk to your doctor first before trying any supplements. Melatonin is a powerful hormone, and researchers are not sure how long-term use may affect your body.

KIDNEY STONES

Relief is just a stone's throw away

Archeologists recently discovered a 7,000 year-old Egyptian mummy with kidney stones, proving this painful condition has plagued people for eons. The good news – after all this time, doctors have learned a little something about who gets them and why.

Your kidneys work like filters, removing waste and extra water from your blood and flushing it all out as urine. They also keep the chemicals, salts, and other substances in your blood carefully balanced. If the minerals and salts become concentrated, they can form crystals in your urine. Between 70 and 90 percent of these crystals wash out of your body unnoticed. But some become large enough to get stuck in your urinary tract on their way out, causing excruciating pain. These large crystals are called stones and there are four main types.

Calcium stones. Most stones are calcium combined with either phosphate or oxalate. More than half of people with kidney stones have an inherited disorder known as hypercalciuria, where their body absorbs too much calcium and flushes out the excess through their kidneys.

Uric acid stones. High-protein foods like red meat and poultry generally pack a lot of purine, which breaks down into uric acid. Your kidneys filter out most of it, but too much in your urine sets the stage for these stones.

Struvite stones. Having a urinary tract infection caused by certain bacteria can lead to these less-common stones.

Cystine stones. These rare, but potentially dangerous, stones develop only in people with an inherited condition that causes high urine levels of cystine, a building block of protein.

White men between the ages of 20 and 50 are most likely to suffer kidney stones, although rates have been rising among obese women. A family history of them also ups your chances. While you can't do much to change your age, gender, or family history, you can adopt a lifestyle proven to cut down on kidney stones.

- Banish that belly. Your risk is greater if you are generally overweight and if you specifically carry extra weight around your middle.
- De-stress. When under pressure, your body releases the hormone vasopressin, which concentrates urine. This might explain why stressful situations seem to trigger kidney stones.
- Swap sides when you snooze. Sleeping in the same position, on the same side, or always on your stomach may increase your risk.
- Keep other conditions under control. High blood pressure, type 2 diabetes, gout, recurrent urinary tract infections, and inflammatory bowel disease (IBD) are all linked to kidney stones.

Amazingly, 70 to 80 percent of people with the most common type of stones, calcium oxalate, can keep them from coming back with simple diet and lifestyle changes – and without resorting to medicine. Have your doctor help you establish a game plan tailored to your type of stone, then read ahead for advice on kicking kidney stones for good.

Water washes away stone risk

Drinking extra water is the single most important thing you can do to fend off any type of kidney stone. You need enough fluids to produce at least two liters – more than eight cups – of pale, watery urine each day. Remember, the point is to dilute your urine, so how much you take in is not as important as how much you turn out. If you're fighting calcium or uric acid stones, aim for 10 glasses of liquids each day, at least half of that water. If you're at risk of cystine stones, you need even more – 16 glasses, or about a gallon, spread evenly throughout the day and night. The key is to drink a little at a time, but drink constantly.

- Have a glass of water with each meal.
- Carry water with you everywhere and sip it regularly. Keep a glass handy around the house, and take bottled water with you while out running errands.
- Try to drink two 8-ounce glasses of water shortly before bedtime.
- Drink more water each time you get up to use the bathroom during the night. You want to prevent your urine from becoming concentrated while you sleep.
- Get more water during hot or dry weather, when you exercise, or if you sweat a lot.

All this extra liquid may not sit well with your body at first. Force yourself to drink it for a couple of months. Your body will get used to the extra fluids, and over time, you'll come to crave them.

Lemonade clobbers calcium crystals

Pucker up. Just half a cup of lemon juice daily could prevent calcium kidney stones. For more than three years, 12 people with recurring calcium oxalate kidney stones drank water flavored with lemon juice. The results were dramatic. They produced fewer stones – a drop of 87 percent – and the stones that did form were smaller. This "lemonade therapy" performed nearly as well as potassium citrate, the first-line medication for this type of kidney stone. It works because lemon juice boosts urine levels of citrate, a chemical that keeps calcium crystals from turning into stones. Too little citrate is a major risk factor for both calcium and uric acid stones.

Lemons share the spotlight with several other stone-fighting juices.

- A small study out of Texas found orange juice increased urinary citrate and prevented uric acid and calcium oxalate from crystallizing. However, some experts warn kidney stone sufferers to avoid OJ since it raises oxalate levels.
- Cranberry juice offers potent protection from urinary tract infections, thereby cutting your risk of struvite stones. But people prone to calcium oxalate and uric acid stones should probably avoid it since it's also rich in oxalates.

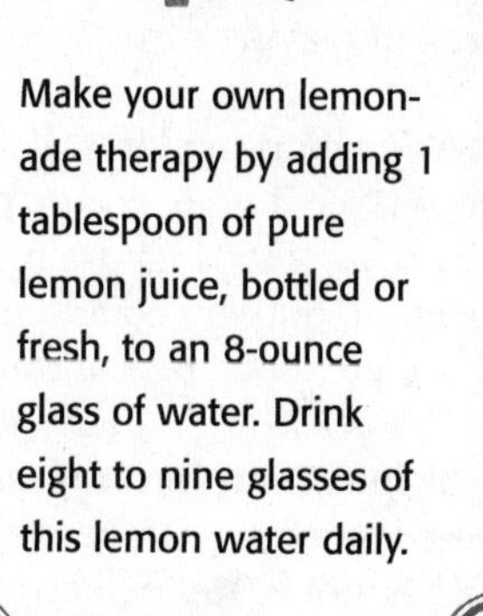

Make your own lemonade therapy by adding 1 tablespoon of pure lemon juice, bottled or fresh, to an 8-ounce glass of water. Drink eight to nine glasses of this lemon water daily.

- In one study, black currant juice made urine less acidic which may prevent uric acid stones from developing.

Eating plan ends pain

Dieters aren't the only ones who should watch what they eat. You can help banish kidney stones for good if you avoid certain foods and make an effort to limit others.

Stay away from added salt. The more sodium you eat, the more calcium in your urine. And remember, when calcium gets too concentrated in urine, it can crystallize into kidney stones. That's why doctors suggest sticking to a low-sodium diet if you are prone to calcium stones. Avoid salting your food, and watch out for "hidden" sources of sodium – fast food, sports drinks, and even canned and frozen foods. Check nutrition labels for sodium content, and try to keep your total intake under 2,000 milligrams a day.

Make meat a smaller part of meals. Protein from meat increases uric acid, calcium, and oxalates in your urine while lowering levels of the protective substance citrate. All that means an increased risk of kidney stones – especially uric acid stones. You can still eat meat, but do it in moderation. Limit yourself to 12 ounces of fish, poultry, beef, or pork a day. That's three servings, each the size of a deck of playing cards.

Ask about oxalates. If you're prone to calcium oxalate kidney stones, see if your doctor recommends watching your oxalate intake. Too many foods naturally contain this compound for you to avoid them all, but you could limit the ones highest in oxalates, such as chocolate, nuts, beans, rhubarb, spinach, beets, and black tea.

Skip certain beverages. Drinking a glass of grapefruit juice daily raised stone risk 44 percent in one eight-year study. Apple juice also makes stones more likely, thanks in part to its oxalates. And research shows caffeine increases the amount of calcium in urine, which can raise calcium stone risk. Some sodas deliver a double whammy, slashing citrate levels in your urine and serving up lots of stone-producing phosphoric acid.

MythBuster: Steer clear of dairy?

Some people think cutting calcium out of your diet will also cut down on calcium stones. Not so. Large studies show people who eat calcium-rich foods enjoy a much lower risk of kidney stones. Dietary calcium seems to tie up oxalates and stop them from passing into your urine and forming stones. The evidence on calcium supplements is mixed, however. Taking up to 1,200 milligrams (mg) a day seems safe, but more than 2,000 mg daily may encourage kidney stones. Keep the mineral from washing out in your urine by taking these supplements with food. In addition, balance all that calcium with plenty of liquids as well as potassium- and phosphate-rich foods like bananas and low-fat milk.

Memory loss

Simple secrets sharpen your recall

Just because you lost your keys doesn't mean you're losing your mind. Everyone forgets things. And the older you get, the more often it seems to happen. Scientists even have a name for it – age-associated memory impairment (AAMI). Rest assured, a moment of forgetfulness is a far cry from Alzheimer's disease (AD).

Scientists used to blame AAMI on the belief that thousands of neurons in your brain die each day. Now they know very few neurons actually die. Instead, they shrink. On top of that, as your body ages, it makes fewer neurotransmitters, the chemical messengers that help brain cells communicate. Add in the fact that blood flow within your brain decreases, and it's no wonder you can't find your keys.

Perhaps most important is your own attitude about getting older. Seniors who believe memory loss is a normal, inevitable part of aging score worse on memory tests, while people who don't harbor such stereotypes do better, sometimes just as well as younger adults. In other words, if you expect your memory to get worse with age, it probably will, maybe because you won't try as hard to remember. Attitude isn't everything, however. The health choices you make have a big impact on your mental sharpness.

Control your cholesterol. You have two types of cholesterol floating around your bloodstream – "good" HDL and "bad" LDL. The goal is to lower your bad and raise your good. In a study of women over 65, higher HDL went hand-in-hand with sharper mental abilities. Cutting LDL, on the other hand, reduces your risk of vascular dementia – memory loss caused by clogged arteries triggering several small, silent strokes.

Banish high blood pressure. When your heart has to work extra hard because of clogged or stiffened arteries, you are at greater risk of vascular dementia. The link between these two conditions may not be fully understood, but it's proven to exist. People with high blood pressure do worse on tests of thinking skills, even if they don't have dementia.

Kick the habit. Smoking doubles your risk of vascular dementia, and smokers over age 65 are almost four times more likely to decline mentally in one year than non- and former-smokers. Experts say smoking may damage the blood vessels in your brain that bring in nutrients.

Small, simple strategies help, too, keeping your memory sharp well into old age. This chapter focuses on preventing age-related memory impairment, not AD. Dementias like Alzheimer's are serious illnesses and should be treated by your doctor.

Mental tricks help you remember

Recalling things isn't as hard as you think. After all, you've spent your whole life doing it. But now you may need a little help. Try these six simple methods to maximize your memory.

Take a deep breath. Anyone who has ever spoken in public or taken a test knows nerves can make your mind go blank. In research studies, some older adults did poorly on timed tests, but when allowed to work at their own pace, these seniors scored as well as young adults. Let go of anxiety before stressful situations through relaxation techniques, and unblock your memory.

Stay focused. Brain research suggests the power to make memories depends largely on your ability to stay alert and interested in what you're learning. Give information your complete attention, block out distractions, and don't try to do two things at once if you want to remember one of them. Multitasking actually impairs your memory.

Use your imagination. Picture yourself doing something in detail and you'll remember to do it in the future. See yourself taking your pills or carrying out the trash. When you meet a new person, link their name to an image that comes to mind. "Jenny" might remind you of a "gem"stone. See the picture in your mind's eye, and you'll be more likely to remember her name the next time you meet.

Talk to yourself. Making comments out loud helps them stick. When you turn off the coffee pot, say "I turned off the coffee pot." The same trick works with names. When you meet someone new, use their name immediately. "Hi, Frank, it's nice to meet you."

Write it down. Even young people make to-do lists. Writing down medication schedules, driving directions, appointments, and phone numbers reinforces them in your memory. Keep a notepad by the phone or in your purse, and hang a calendar in a visible spot where you can easily refer to it.

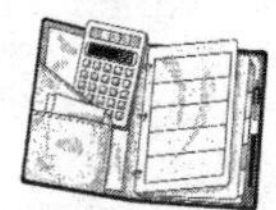

Establish a routine. Habits come almost without thinking because they are part of your daily routine. Make any act a habit by setting up an easy-to-follow schedule. For instance, take medications with the same meal or after the same TV show every day.

Common prescriptions cloud your thinking

The most common cause of memory loss is not Alzheimer's disease. It's a reaction to prescription, and even over-the-counter, medications. Older adults are more susceptible to drug side effects and interactions because they take more medications than most young people – an average of five prescription plus three over-the-counter medicines. Plus, aging slows down how your body processes drugs, so they stay in your system longer.

You can take steps to prevent this, however. Pay attention when you begin a new medication. Take note of how you feel, and see your doctor if you notice worrisome symptoms like cloudy thinking or forgetfulness. Never stop taking your medicine on your own, but put all your medications, both prescription and over-the-counter, in a bag and take it with you to the doctor's office. Be sure to bring the original bottles and dosage instructions. She'll go through them to see if any could be causing your memory loss. Simply changing a prescription or adjusting the dosage could get you back to normal. These popular medications are a few of the drugs linked to memory problems.

- alprazolam (Xanax)
- aspirin
- atenolol (Tenormin)
- cephalexin (Biocef, Keflex)
- cimetidine (Tagamet HB)
- ciprofloxacin (Cipro)
- clonazepam (Klonopin)
- codeine
- cyclobenzaprine (Flexeril)
- diazepam (Valium)
- diphenhydramine (Benadryl)
- hydrocodone
- ibuprofen (Advil, Motrin)
- lorazepam (Ativan)
- metoprolol (Lopressor)
- naproxen (Naprosyn)
- prednisone (Deltasone)
- propoxyphene (Darvon-N)
- pseudoephedrine (Claritin-D)
- ranitidine (Zantac 75)

Amazing brain foods outwit old age

Scientists may never discover an anti-aging pill, but you can keep your brain young and your memory sharp by eating any number of convenient and delicious foods. No drug side effects, just balanced nutrition – what could be better or simpler?

Bite into an apple. Chances are, this "miracle" memory improver is already in your kitchen, and you're going to want to grab one – or two – right away. Apples may slow mental decline by boosting brain levels of acetylcholine, a chemical that enables brain cells to communicate. Better communication seems to mean enhanced memory. So far, experts have only conducted research on animals, but they say a daily dose of two cups of apple juice or two to three apples made a noticeable difference. Shop for apple juice without added sugar to cut down extra calories.

Eat those veggies. Getting your greens may be the best thing you can do to keep a younger brain, says a new study from the Rush Institute for Healthy Aging. Over the course of six years, people 65 and older who ate three or more servings of vegetables a day slowed their mental decline by 40 percent, compared to seniors eating only one serving daily.

Angle for more fish. Would you like to be as mentally sharp as you were three or four years ago? Then add fish to your weekly menu. Past studies have linked eating fish to lower risks of stroke and dementia. Now new research says it could protect you from age-related memory loss, slowing mental decline by 10 to 13 percent.

Become a berry-picker. Fruits like blueberries and strawberries pack large amounts of polyphenols, natural compounds that counteract age-related damage in the brain. Based on rat studies, these polyphenols also improve memory and learning skills. Toss a handful of berries onto your cereal or whip some into a smoothie, then go dazzle someone with all the things you can remember.

Ginseng gets your mind in gear

It's an ancient Chinese secret claiming to keep your mind and body young into advanced years – and researchers say it works. Several studies give Asian (Panax) ginseng a thumbs up, stating it improves brain function, including reaction time, learning, concentration, math, and logic skills. People healthy or ill, young or old seem to benefit from this herb, at least in the short-term. And in Europe, ginseng is used as an all-around feel-good remedy, said to bolster your health when you're under stress plus perk up mood, vigor, and your sense of well-being.

Most studies have tested 200 milligrams of ginseng extract daily, or 0.5 to 2 grams of dry root. If you choose the extract, look for one made with 4 to 7 percent ginsenosides, the active ingredients. Experts generally recommend using the herb for two to three weeks, then taking a break for a week or two. It seems safe and rarely leads to side effects, although women who have had breast cancer should not take ginseng since it may stimulate the growth of breast cancer cells. Also, if you are diabetic or on a blood-thinning medication, like warfarin (Coumadin), talk to your doctor before trying this supplement.

Gentle workouts 'jog' your memory

That couch potato lifestyle could be draining your brain. A study of elderly men found their thinking abilities declined as they became less active. That may be in part because what's good for the heart is good for the brain. Regular exercise improves thinking ability and lowers your risk for age-related mental decline. And

Move & groove: good for your brain

Past research pointed to classical music, especially Mozart, as the ultimate brain booster. But newer studies suggest the best melodies for a mental pick-me-up are simply ones you enjoy. So, go ahead and indulge your fondness for jazz or your secret love of show tunes. Want to improve your mental skills even more? Learning to play a musical instrument may improve your ability to read, work with numbers, remember words, and concentrate – plus generally raise your IQ.

And don't feel shy about doing a little two-step. Dancing combines music and movement for a one-two workout – mental because you have to remember the dance steps, physical because it gets your heart pumping. In one study, seniors who danced frequently were 76 percent less likely to develop dementia.

exercises that get your heart pumping, like aerobics, literally make your brain grow.

Brisk walking may be all you need. Women who walked at least an hour and a half each week enjoyed sharper minds than those who walked less than 40 minutes a week. Aim for around 30 minutes of moderate activity most days of the week – yard work, swimming, walking, bowling, or something else you enjoy. Don't do the same routine day after day, though. Research from Johns Hopkins University finds a variety of activities really is the spice of life, offering much more protection from dementia.

Restful sleep restores your mind

Boost your memory and sharpen your mind overnight just by getting a little shuteye. Sleep is essential for spot-on recollection and clear thinking because, at night, while your body rests, your brain busily organizes memories and stores them more efficiently. They even become more permanent. During sleep, you also strengthen the connections between brain cells and between different parts of your brain. This keeps your memories, skills, and other knowledge from eroding over time. Getting your forty winks can even help you recover seemingly "lost" memories.

Forgetfulness isn't surprising given that sleep problems become more common with age. Improve your chances of a full night's rest by going to bed and waking up at the same time every day; avoiding heavy meals right before bed; and moving the TV, computer, and other distractions out of the bedroom. Read more on resting well in the *Insomnia* chapter.

B vitamins safeguard your brain

Control the amount of homocysteine in your body and you control your risk of impaired memory. This amino acid injures your arteries and encourages blood clots. The result is an increased risk of stroke. And you know strokes are a major cause of mental decline. When one group of seniors experienced out-of-control homocysteine levels, *The New England Journal of Medicine* reported they were twice as likely to develop vascular dementia or Alzheimer's within eight years.

While you naturally have more homocysteine in your blood as you get older, you're protected if you get enough folate, vitamin B6, and vitamin B12 in your diet – since these vitamins break down homocysteine. Some experts recommend taking a multivitamin to prevent deficiency, but B supplements can't always perk up your memory. Long-term vitamin deficiencies may have already done irreversible damage. That means it's especially important to build B-rich foods into your regular diet early on and eat them throughout your life.

- Vitamin B6 is abundant in whole grains, fruits, dark leafy greens, and legumes.
- Meat, fish, dairy, and eggs are fantastic sources of vitamin B12.
- Get an extra boost of folate from dark leafy greens, legumes, seeds, and enriched breads and cereals.

Homespun remedies

Sweet-scented rosemary aids memory

"There's rosemary, that's for remembrance; pray, love, remember." Shakespeare's Ophelia wasn't the first to think rosemary could help you remember. The idea took hold in ancient Greece. Anxious students looking for an academic edge wore sprigs of rosemary in their hair in the belief it aided memory.

Motion Sickness

Easy ways to enjoy the ride

Traveling should be about exploring new places, visiting friends and family, and appreciating the scenery along the way. But when you suffer from motion sickness, you spend your trip fighting off nausea instead.

Like a powerful army, motion sickness can strike by land, air, or sea. It starts with a feeling of "stomach awareness" and warmth. You feel nauseous, become pale, sweat, salivate, and eventually vomit or retch. You may also feel dizzy, fatigued, or depressed and experience headaches.

Motion sickness happens when your brain receives contradictory information from your eyes, inner ear – which controls balance – and muscle sensors. For instance, if you're reading a book in a car, your eyes see a stationary page with words while your body feels the car's movement, leaving your brain with conflicting information. A rocking boat, a winding road, turbulence on a flight, and amusement park rides can all trigger motion sickness. You don't even need to be moving – flight simulators and video games can have the same effect.

About one-third of the population experiences motion sickness. It affects women more often than men, but becomes less of a problem as you age. The peak years for motion sickness are ages 3 through 12 – but it can strike anyone.

Folk remedies for motion sickness include taping your navel, placing a piece of stationery on your chest, wearing a paper bag over your head, tying a red string around your waist, putting an onion or raw potato in your pocket, or stuffing a dollar bill down your shirt. But these odd remedies might just make you feel foolish and queasy.

Both over-the-counter and prescription drugs can help. You can find antihistamines, like dimenhydrinate (Dramamine) or meclizine (Bonine or Dramamine II), at your local drugstore. The prescription drug scopolamine, available as a skin patch called Transderm Scop, may be even more effective because it provides a steady stream of medicine. Just remember that these drugs come with the risk of side effects, like drowsiness, dry mouth, and blurred vision.

There are also plenty of simple, self-help steps you can take to prevent motion sickness that don't involve paper bags, red string, raw potatoes, or drugs.

- Choose your seat wisely. Sit in the front seat of a car, over the wings on an airplane, or mid-ship on a boat.
- Drive rather than be a passenger. It will help you anticipate the twists and turns of the road.
- Get plenty of fresh air. Avoid strong odors, such as smoke, cologne, or food.
- Don't read or watch videos.
- Keep your head still. Use a headrest and lie back for maximum comfort.

Homespun remedies

Newspapers deliver surprising benefits

Stop the presses! Keeping a newspaper in your car may help fight motion sickness – as long as you don't try to read it. Simply take a whiff instead. For some people, the smell of newsprint provides relief when they're feeling carsick. Try this unusual remedy next time you hit the road. You may find that, like an ace reporter, you have a nose for news.

- Face forward and focus on the horizon. Keep your eyes on a fixed, stable object rather than moving ones.

Ginger gets to the root of the problem

You know drugs can prevent motion sickness, but their potential side effects worry you. So tread gingerly – and reach for some ginger. This herbal remedy provides cheap, effective relief.

Experts remain unsure why ginger helps, but they believe it acts directly on the stomach. However it works, ginger has some research to back it up. In one study of 80 new sailors who hadn't yet found their sea legs, those who took ginger experienced less vomiting and cold sweats than those who took a placebo, or dummy pill. A recent Taiwanese study also found that ginger reduces nausea and helps prevent and treat motion sickness.

Other studies of ginger have reported less positive results – but if you're prone to motion sickness, it can't hurt to give this common folk remedy a try.

You can find ginger in several forms, including powder, capsules, candied, crystallized, or tea. For best results, take 500 milligrams of powdered ginger root about a half-hour before traveling. Repeat the dose every four hours as needed. Two one-inch squares of candied ginger should also do the trick.

Breathe your way to relief

You're stuck on a swaying boat or shaky plane. You feel that familiar queasiness coming on. Don't panic. Just breathe. Simply breathing the right way can help ward off motion sickness. Studies show controlled breathing, a technique that focuses on breathing gently and regularly through your nose, helps people overcome motion sickness. Yet, rapid, shallow breaths can make things worse.

While controlled breathing works only about half as well as drugs, it costs absolutely nothing and comes with zero side effects.

Pressure pushes nausea away

Motion sickness may affect your stomach and head, but to find relief, it's all in the wrist. Thanks to a technique called acupressure, queasy travelers have the solution to motion sickness right at their fingertips. Simply applying pressure to a certain spot on your wrist may be enough to make you feel better.

Like acupuncture but without the needles, acupressure uses finger pressure on specific body sites to promote healing. The point that helps with nausea and motion sickness, called P6, is located two finger-widths below the crease of your wrist in the groove between the two tendons that begin at the base of your palm.

In addition to pushing on this spot yourself, you can also buy special wristbands – with brand names like Sea-Band, Acuband, and Queaz-Away – that apply pressure. Some studies show these wristbands, available in drugstores or on the Internet, can be effective in managing nausea. In fact, the FDA has approved them as remedies for motion sickness. But other studies have found no benefit from wristbands.

Acupressure is not for everyone. People with brittle bones should beware. Wristbands may also present risks. Those with batteries that create a small electric charge, like ReliefBand, may cause a rash or interfere with pacemakers.

Smart choices settle your stomach

Unless your trip is to the electric chair, you don't want your last meal before traveling to be a large one. A big, greasy meal may sound yummy, but once you get moving, you could regret it. What you put in your belly before and during traveling helps determine whether you get sick or not. To prevent motion sickness, avoid the following things, which can aggravate nausea.

- alcohol
- smoking
- dairy products
- high-calorie, high-protein foods
- salty, greasy, and spicy foods
- strong-smelling or strong-tasting foods

On the other hand, you can make smart food choices and serve up an extra portion of protection. Try these strategies for a smooth trip.

- Eat small, light meals or snacks low in calories.
- Munch on dry crackers or sip a carbonated beverage if you feel sick.
- Choose low-fat, starchy foods.
- Use caffeine to counteract the drowsiness caused by drugs.

Kitchen cures for queasiness

Some travelers pack light, living out of a backpack for months at a time. Others pack everything but the kitchen sink. Definitely leave the sink at home, but consider packing some of these motion sickness remedies you can find in your kitchen.

Cardamom. This spice has antinausea powers and may stimulate digestion. One traditional remedy involved boiling roasted cardamom seeds along with betel nuts to form a drink to treat nausea and indigestion.

> Put motion sickness on ice. Applying a cold pack to your forehead may help soothe your stomach during a rough trip.

Lemon. Folk remedies for seasickness include eating a whole lemon or sucking its juice. Just the scent of lemon may also soothe nausea. The American Cancer Society recommends eating foods with pleasant smells, like lemon drops or mints, to control nausea.

Peppermint. Some herbalists recommend the combination of black horehound and peppermint to treat the nausea that comes with motion sickness. Peppermint, which gets its power from its essential oils, has been used to treat nausea, vomiting, and dizziness. A soothing cup of peppermint tea may calm your upset stomach.

Mouth sores

Take the bite out of cankers and cold sores

They seem to come out of nowhere, those pesky little sores in your mouth that hurt like heck and make eating no fun. What can you do about them? Start by figuring out what kind of mouth sore is making you miserable, so you can decide how to treat it. Here are two of the most common.

Canker sores. These small, white ulcers outlined in red are often quite painful. It's unclear exactly what causes them, but stress, eating certain foods, or taking some drugs might bring them on. They are not contagious, and they usually disappear within two weeks.

Try these tips to make things more bearable while your canker sore heals.

- Stay away from hot, spicy, or acidic foods.
- Try to relax and avoid extra stress in your life.
- Shun aspirin, which can irritate a canker sore with its acidity.

Over-the-counter drugs won't cure canker sores, but they can mask the pain to make eating and drinking more comfortable. Oragel cuts the pain with benzocaine, while Canker Cover contains menthol to soothe your gums.

Cold sores. These are sometimes called fever blisters. Unlike canker sores, which are found inside the mouth, most cold sores are on the outside of the lips or skin near the mouth. The herpes simplex virus causes cold sores, and once you've had the virus you're apt to get these little reminders all your life. The herpes virus is contagious, so don't touch someone else's cold sore.

Most fever blisters go away within a couple weeks, but they can be pretty ugly. Here are some ways to keep them under control.

- Keep the cold sore clean and dry, perhaps with cornstarch.
- Don't touch the sore, and keep your hands and nails clean.
- Try an ice pack to block the pain and keep cold sores from coming back. Ice can suppress the herpes virus.
- Wear sun block or lip balm with sunscreen. Studies show sunlight can trigger a herpes outbreak.

Aspirin can help with the pain, and it might even make your cold sore heal more quickly. You may need a prescription antiviral drug if you have a severe outbreak of the herpes virus.

Kiss away cold sores with natural relief

You might be able to stick with nature's treatments instead of drugs if your cold sores aren't too bothersome. Many traditional remedies, like goldenseal and garlic, have not been proven to work. But a few home therapies have the blessing of scientific evidence.

Simple home brew calms canker sores

Next time canker sore pain interferes with eating, try this cheap kitchen remedy. Mix a spoonful of baking soda in warm salt water, and use it as a mouth rinse several times a day. Baking soda battles the acidity around the sore, while salt causes a mild chemical burn on the skin's surface to speed healing. You'll be free of pain and enjoying your meals again in no time.

Aloe vera gel is an antiviral. The gooey stuff from inside the leaves of this hardy plant has many uses, including killing viruses and promoting healing. Cream containing aloe vera was found to work against the herpes simplex virus in the genital area, ending the virus outbreak of most people in the study. More research may show whether aloe vera works just as well on fever blisters, caused by the same virus.

Honey hampers the herpes virus. As simple as it sounds, rubbing some pure honey on your cold sores can make them heal faster and hurt less. Researchers found honey worked better and with fewer side effects than one popular prescription cold sore drug. Honey is famous for killing bacteria, and it's shown to battle some viruses as well. It also contains nutrients like vitamin C, vitamin E, and zinc – all known to knock out the herpes virus.

Lemon balm is popular in Europe. Studies show lemon balm cream can reduce cold sore symptoms, probably because the tannins and caffeic acid it contains kill viruses. It's a tried-and-true remedy for inflammation caused by other skin problems like insect bites and skin irritation.

Balanced diet blasts fever blisters

You know how important it is to eat right, but what exactly should you eat to avoid a cold sore? It's all about balance.

MythBuster: Can zinc zap cold sores?

The mineral zinc keeps the herpes virus from reproducing, which can end a rash of cold sores or genital herpes and prevent future outbreaks. But it only works with creams and watery solutions of zinc sulfate or zinc oxide-glycine. The zinc cream you buy over the counter has zinc oxide, which doesn't release enough of the mineral to help. Look for zinc creams specially formulated to combat cold sores.

Keep amino acids in proportion. Your body needs several amino acids – the building blocks of protein – to survive. More than 30 years ago, researchers began looking at the amino acids lysine and arginine to see how their balance might affect the virus that causes cold sores. Here's what they found.

- Go heavy on lysine. It seems that having lots of lysine in your cells makes it hard for the herpes virus to reproduce. Studies have shown that taking a daily supplement of lysine while eating less arginine can make outbreaks of cold sores less frequent. The best dose of lysine, sometimes called l-lysine, is not known, but 500 to 3,000 milligrams (mg) per day seems to work. Aim for more lysine in your diet from legumes or animal proteins, and boil or poach meats rather than grilling or frying them.
- Take it easy on arginine. Having lots of arginine around helps the herpes virus, bringing on more cold sore bouts. Stay away from chocolate, nuts, and seeds, which can have a lot of arginine.

Vanquish cold sores with vitamin C. You know this wonder nutrient can prevent scurvy and possibly the common cold, but did you know it helps fight cold sores? One study showed that adding 600 mg to your diet every day helps beef up your immune system enough to scare away a herpes attack quickly. Add more vitamin-C-rich foods to your diet, like oranges and red peppers, or consider taking a supplement.

Toothpaste ingredient irritates mouth

Your toothpaste may be the culprit if you suffer from repeated bouts with cold sores or canker sores. Sodium lauryl sulphate (SLS), a common additive that makes toothpaste frothy and foamy, can irritate gums. Researchers in Finland compared toothpaste with and without SLS on the gums of 20 volunteers, finding the SLS toothpaste caused more irritation. Aside from discomfort, this irritation also raises the risk of infection. Look for a toothpaste without sodium lauryl sulphate on the ingredient list like Rembrandt Canker Sore Toothpaste.

NAIL PROBLEMS

Get a grip on unsightly nails

Beautiful fingernails have long been a symbol of femininity and gentility. Some cultures see long, carefully groomed nails as a sign of high status, since most people who work for a living put wear and tear on their nails. Depending on where you live, having dirt under your nails can be a sign of hard work or poor grooming. In the point of view of humorist and actor Will Rogers, "What the country needs is dirtier fingernails and cleaner minds."

Nails are also functional, helping you pick up small items and protecting your fingers and toes. Some jobs and hobbies require groomed nails, like the string-plucking fingers of a classical guitarist or the needle-pushing finger of a quilter who shuns a thimble.

A doctor can get a sense of your health and nutrition by checking both the condition of your nails and the color and blood supply in your nail bed – the flesh you see when you look through the clear part of your fingernail or toenail. Ingrown toenails, brittle fingernails, and nail fungus are common among adults.

With a bit of attention to what you eat and how you treat your fingers and toes, you can nail down a perfect 20 – 10 lovely fingernails and 10 well-groomed toenails.

Biotin battles brittle nails

Aging, too much time in water, contact with harsh chemicals, or other stresses can make your nails brittle – easily broken, lined or ridged, thin, and dry. Poor nutrition can also cause this condition. If you don't get enough iron, vitamins A and C, zinc, omega-3 fatty acids, and biotin in your diet, your nails will suffer. However, research has not found that taking supplements of these nutrients can help your nails – except for biotin.

Biotin, a B-complex vitamin, helps your body form keratin, which makes up hair and nails. Researchers tested 2.5 milligrams of biotin each day for six months on people with brittle nails. This dose improved the nail health and growth of 63 percent of the people who took it. Since this is a large dose, check with your doctor before trying biotin therapy. You can also get more biotin in your diet from milk, egg yolks, fish, and whole grains.

MythBuster: Can gelatin strengthen nails?

Do you recall watching your mother dissolve an envelope of unflavored gelatin in water and down the gritty drink every day? Even today, many people believe drinking gelatin will strengthen their nails. Unfortunately, it's just an old wives' tale. Early marketing of gelatin suggested this animal byproduct would provide protein to help grow strong nails. Your body needs a balanced diet, including enough protein and essential vitamins and minerals, to produce the keratin that makes up healthy nails. But drinking gelatin won't give your nails extra help.

Simple ways to defeat common nail woes

Some people have no trouble growing long nails. In fact, according to *Guinness World Records*, the world's longest nails belong to a woman in Utah. She grew one thumbnail to more than 31 inches long. But most people have to work a little harder to keep their nails healthy and looking great.

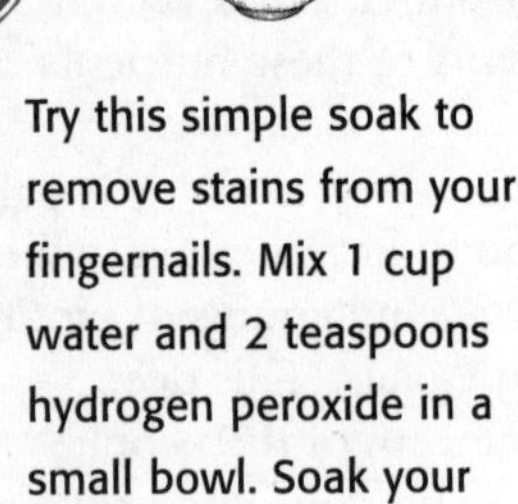

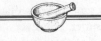

Try this simple soak to remove stains from your fingernails. Mix 1 cup water and 2 teaspoons hydrogen peroxide in a small bowl. Soak your fingertips for about 10 minutes. If the stains are not completely gone, scrub under your nails with a soft brush. Then rinse, dry, and apply moisturizer. If you prefer a natural option, rub a lemon wedge on your nail tips to make them whiter.

Water loss is the main cause of brittle nails. Too much time washing dishes or exposure to harsh soaps or chemicals can sap the moisture from your nails. If you must use chemicals, shield your nails by wearing cotton gloves inside rubber gloves. Protecting your nails with polish can help, but don't use polish remover too often. The acetone in most removers takes away even more moisture from your nails. Use a nail moisturizer with petrolatum, mineral oil, or alpha hydroxy acids to keep nails supple.

The best way to deal with ingrown toenails is to avoid getting them. Trim your toenails straight across rather than curved, and don't cut them too short. Don't wear tight or narrow shoes that crowd your toes. If you have a painful ingrown toenail, give it plenty of room by wearing sandals.

To relieve the discomfort, soak your feet in warm salt water, then push back the softened skin around your ingrown nail. Place a small wisp of cotton under the sharp edge to stop it from digging into your skin. Insert a clean piece of cotton every day until your nail grows past this tender area. To prevent an infection, apply antibiotic ointment to the cotton. If your ingrown toenail becomes infected, see your doctor.

Tea tree oil tough on nail fungus

Several types of fungus can invade your nails, especially if you are older or have diabetes or circulatory problems. The fungus that causes athlete's foot can attack your toenails, and you're more likely to get it if you play sports or wear tight shoes. Men often get fungus on their toenails, while women tend to get it on fingernails.

If you have a nail fungus, you'll probably notice one or more nails with cloudy white or yellowish spots. Nails with fungus usually get thicker and can be crumbly and flaky. As the fungus grows, it can produce waste, which collects under your nail to make it grow up instead of out. Your nail may eventually loosen and even fall off.

You don't have to suffer in silence. If you have a problem on your toes, start with the same steps that can banish athlete's foot – keep your feet dry and cool. Some people say vinegar treatment works, but researchers haven't found it useful for nail fungus.

For a mild case of nail fungus, you can try tea tree oil, a natural antifungal. One study showed tea tree oil worked as well as clotrimazole, a common antifungal cream, at clearing up toenail fungus after six months of use. People in the study used tea tree oil every day at full strength, which can cause problems if you are sensitive or allergic to it.

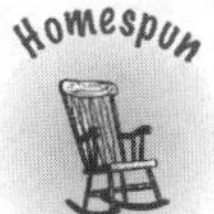

Cough remedy rubs out nail fungus

Nurses at a foot-care clinic made an interesting discovery. Some of their patients were using Vicks VapoRub to treat nail fungus, and it seemed to work. The nurses suggested this remedy to other patients and kept track of the results. Many people who tried the throat rub didn't come back for checkups, but most of those who kept at it had success. So researchers tested the theory in the lab using a different brand, Meijer's Medicated Chest Rub. This product killed the types of fungus that most commonly infect toenails. Camphor, eucalyptus oil, and menthol are the active ingredients in both brands. You'll need to rub on the ointment once a day for several months until the fungal infection clears up.

You'll need to see a doctor if you have a more serious nail fungus problem. Ointments and other surface remedies have trouble reaching the fungus under the nail, so you may need to take a prescription drug, like terbinafine (Lamisil) or itraconazole (Sporanox), to kill the fungus. You'll have to take these medications for a long time – likely for months – and some can damage your liver or heart. Ask your doctor about a new drug, ciclopirox (Penlac), which you paint on your nails like a polish.

Sidestep nail salon dangers

Having a manicure or pedicure at a salon feels like a luxury, but beware of hidden hazards. Tools or footbaths contaminated with bacteria, viruses, or fungi can cause a serious infection. Follow these safety rules to avoid a problem.

- Make sure the salon's tools are disinfected between uses. This includes whirlpool footbaths, which should be bleached regularly.
- Buy your own tools, like emery boards that can't be sterilized, and bring them to your salon appointment.
- Forget about shaving your legs before a pedicure. Small nicks or cuts on your skin can let in bacteria from dirty water.
- Don't let a technician cut your cuticles or razor off calluses. These sharp tools can damage healthy skin and make way for harmful invaders.
- Look for your manicurist's state cosmetology license, which should be on view.

Another salon danger is an allergic reaction. Most states have banned the poisonous chemical methyl methacrylate (MMA) from use in salons since it can cause nail deformities, infections, and allergic reactions. But some inexpensive salons may still use it because it's cheap and makes acrylic nails strong. Some people are allergic to other chemicals, like formaldehyde, often found in nail hardeners.

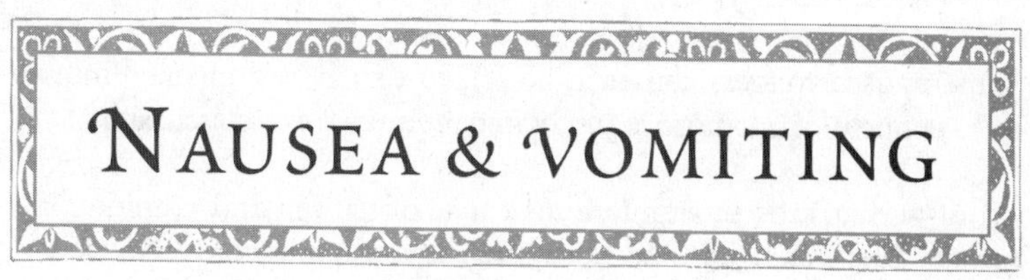

NAUSEA & VOMITING

Super ways to calm an agitated stomach

You'll ease that queasy feeling if you make a poultice of ginger, cloves, cinnamon, black pepper, cayenne, and honey and apply it to the pit of your stomach. At least that's what an old Arkansas folk remedy claims. But if you're nauseated, you probably feel too ill to do that much work. Instead, arm yourself with the latest information about nausea so you'll know when to treat it yourself and when to call your doctor.

When you are nauseated, you feel like you are on the verge of vomiting. You may also have fever, sweating, chills, weakness, cramps, dry heaves, and an upset stomach. You might not realize it but nausea and vomiting are key defenders against germs, irritants, and other substances that can harm your body.

For example, if some troublemaker triggers enough stomach acid to irritate your stomach lining, your stomach can send chemical messengers, like dopamine and serotonin, to get help. These messengers head straight for your brain's vomiting center. Their arrival can trigger nausea. If your brain's vomiting center detects enough danger, it also sends orders to your diaphragm, respiratory system, digestive system, and muscles to make vomiting happen.

Nausea and vomiting are often symptoms of health problems, such as migraines or stomach flu. Other causes of the "Big Queasy" include overeating, motion sickness, dizziness, stress, or disturbing smells or sights, like seeing someone else vomit. But remember – nausea and vomiting can also be side effects of medication, so check the label and ask your doctor about switching to another drug.

Some nausea triggers can even be serious, such as a blocked intestine, peptic ulcer, exposure to chemical toxins, or a concussion.

But perhaps the most infamous cause of nausea and vomiting in recent years has been food poisoning. It can happen anytime you accidentally eat food contaminated by viruses, parasites, pesticides, or certain bacteria, like *E. coli.* Although the germs behind food poisoning are usually most plentiful in eggs, meat, poultry, and milk, spinach was the source of a recent *E. coli* outbreak.

If you get food poisoning, you will probably have severe nausea, diarrhea, fever, and chills. You might get them within hours of eating tainted food or several days later.

Fortunately, most people recover in a few days from food poisoning, and you may recover even more quickly from other cases of nausea and vomiting. But if you stay sick and don't know what caused it, see your doctor. Otherwise, use these tips to help you feel better.

When nausea spells danger

Call your doctor immediately or go to the emergency room if you develop any of these symptoms along with nausea or vomiting.

- fever of 101 degrees Fahrenheit or higher
- rapid breathing or pulse
- vomit or stool that's bloody or resembles coffee grounds
- agonizing headache or stiff neck
- projectile vomiting or severe abdominal pain
- vomiting for more than two days
- go 24 hours without keeping liquids down
- have diarrhea for more than three days
- signs of dehydration, like excessive thirst, dizziness, dry mouth, dark-yellow urine, or little or no urine

- Rest and drink lots of liquids as soon as you can keep them down to prevent dehydration. If you are vomiting, take small, frequent sips. Start with clear drinks, such as water and apple juice. Avoid teas, carbonated or caffeinated drinks, sports drinks, and acidic juices like orange juice.
- Try antacids or over-the-counter bismuth solutions, like Pepto-Bismol.
- Add bland foods slowly as your symptoms dwindle. Begin with the BRAT diet – bananas, rice, applesauce, and toast. Then add easily digested foods, like broth, gelatin, saltine crackers, cooked cereals, or plain bread, to ease back into solid foods. Avoid high-fiber foods and dairy products for several days, as well as caffeine, alcohol, fatty or spicy foods, aspirin, and other nonsteroidal anti-inflammatory drugs (NSAIDs).

Herbal teas bring gentle relief

Two herbs beloved by the ancient Greeks and Romans could help ease the queasies. These herbs – lemon balm and chamomile – can soothe your nausea by calming spasms in your digestive tract.

To make a cup of lightly scented lemon balm tea, steep up to 3 teaspoons of the leaves in 8 ounces of boiling water for six to 10 minutes. Strain and sip slowly.

If you can't find lemon balm, buy chamomile tea bags from the grocery store instead. Just remember, you probably should skip lemon balm if you have glaucoma or thyroid problems. On the other hand, if you're allergic to ragweed, chrysanthemums, celery, or onions, you may be allergic to chamomile, too. That's when lemon balm is your best choice.

Powerful spice offers serious protection

Ginger is not just for motion sickness. This old-fashioned remedy can help reduce the nausea and vomiting that often follow surgery, says a review of recent research. Many health professionals also suspect ginger might ease nausea and vomiting from other causes.

Ginger blocks nausea like the goaltender in a soccer game blocks balls. Here's how it works. Possible danger signals, like too much stomach acid, cause your stomach to send a chemical messenger called serotonin to your brain. If serotonin reaches your brain's vomiting center, it may start issuing orders to set off vomiting. But, like that goaltender, ginger blocks serotonin, so it can't get its message to your vomiting center. And that can be enough to prevent or ease nausea.

If you have upcoming surgery and would like to try ginger, ask your doctor first. Ginger has blood-thinning powers that could cause dangerous bleeding during surgery. Studies suggest taking a gram of ginger an hour before surgery. Ask your doctor if ginger is safe for you. Keep in mind the hospital might not let you take ginger without your doctor's permission.

Even though ginger might also be effective against other kinds of nausea, get your doctor's OK before you test it. Large doses could interact with insulin and antacids, irritate your stomach, or increase the effects of blood-thinning drugs, like aspirin and warfarin. What's more, people with gallbladder disease should never take ginger.

If your doctor gives you a "green light" for ginger, try candied ginger or make a tea. Grate a level tablespoon of fresh ginger. Combine it with 8 ounces of water in a tightly covered saucepan, bring to a boil, and simmer for about nine minutes on low heat. Let cool for five minutes before drinking. If ginger causes burping or burning in your throat, talk to your doctor about ginger capsules.

Wristbands quiet queasiness without drugs

The drugstore wristbands famed for fighting motion sickness may banish other kinds of nausea, too. These queasy-relief bands are based on the ancient Chinese art of acupressure, which is similar to acupuncture but without the scary needles.

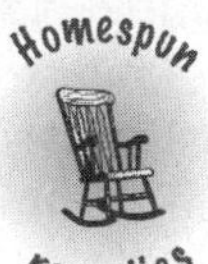

Cold cloth cuts queasiness

For gentle relief, wet a washcloth with cold water, wring it out, and rest it on your throat or the back of your neck. When the cloth no longer feels cold, dampen it with a fresh round of chilly water and reapply.

Each band contains a bead used to stimulate the acupressure point near your inner wrist. New research suggests this may affect the electrical activity in the muscles of your digestive tract. That electrical activity gets fouled up during nausea and vomiting, causing your muscles to act differently than they should. But scientists suspect stimulating the acupressure point on your forearm may help those digestive tract muscles get back to normal.

If you'd like to try this ancient Chinese secret, pick up a pair of Sea-Bands or similar bands at the drugstore and follow the directions carefully.

Breathing trick blows away 'unsettled' feeling

Sometimes an inexpensive, old-fashioned remedy beats one that's more advanced – and more expensive. That's what happened when researchers studied aromatherapy for after-surgery nausea. They pitted two different scented wipes against an unscented "placebo" wipe. But, to their surprise, the unscented wipe fought nausea just as well as the scented pads. The researchers say the unscented cloths worked because they helped the surgery patients practice controlled breathing.

Controlled breathing differs from regular breathing because you use your diaphragm instead of your upper chest muscles and shoulders. In fact, some experts think that's the key. Your brain needs your diaphragm and other organs involved in breathing to help make vomiting happen. But if those organs are busy with controlled breathing, it might interfere with the process needed for nausea and vomiting. Other experts point out that your brain's vomiting center is close to the part of your brain that manages breathing. They suspect the breathing center interferes with the vomiting center activities.

If you'd like to try controlled breathing, find your diaphragm first. Press your hand just below your breastbone and give a little cough. Your diaphragm will push against your palm. Leave your hand over your diaphragm and breathe in slowly through your nose. Then breathe out through your mouth. If you feel your diaphragm move each time and your breaths are unhurried, you're practicing controlled breathing. This simple, drug-free remedy may be all you need to make your nausea fade away.

Quick vinegar fix fights food poisoning

You've just finished your spinach salad when the news channel announces a nationwide spinach recall because of dangerous *E. coli* bacteria. Don't panic. Instead, mix 2 teaspoons of apple cider vinegar into a glass of mineral water and drink up. This might kill the bacteria before they can make you sick.

10 hot tips to stop food poisoning cold

You can help prevent *E. coli* food poisoning in ground beef and burgers just by adding 1 tablespoon of dried plum puree per pound of ground beef. But that's not all. Beat back food poisoning with these 10 terrific tricks.

- Add 3 to 5 teaspoons of garlic powder to every 2 pounds of ground beef.

- Keep baked potatoes steaming hot until you serve them. Bacteria breed under the foil wrappers.

- Combine a half-cup to 1 cup of tasty chopped onions with each pound of ground beef before grilling to prevent poisoning from *Salmonella.*

- Refrigerate leftovers, perishables, and prepared food quickly. Never leave them at room temperature for more than two hours.
- Cook food to at least 160 degrees Fahrenheit, including leafy greens.
- Reheat cooked food to at least 165 degrees Fahrenheit.
- Use your fridge, microwave, or cold running water to defrost food instead of your kitchen counter.
- Clean your hands, utensils, and cutting boards between foods, especially when those foods are raw meat, poultry, fish, shellfish, or eggs.
- Discard the outermost leaves on heads of lettuce and cabbage.
- Wash any plate that held raw meat, poultry, fish, or shellfish in hot, soapy water before you use it again.

Sugary drinks soothe stomachs best

Your doctor told you to take a "phosphorylated carbohydrate syrup," like Emetrol, but you don't have any in the house. Don't worry. Melt small bites of Popsicle in your mouth or slowly sip clear liquids, like cranberry juice, apple juice, grape juice, Hi-C or Kool-Aid. Like Emetrol, these sugary drinks help you stay hydrated, coat your stomach, and give you energy to recover. And, for reasons doctors don't understand, they also help ease nausea. If you have diabetes, ask your doctor for another remedy. Otherwise, try this easy remedy and see how much it helps.

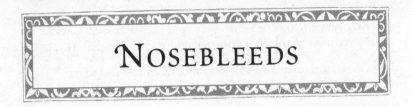

NOSEBLEEDS

Soothing strategies staunch the flow

Most people panic at a nosebleed – whether it's simply a trickle or a terrifying flood. The fact is, nearly all of them look worse than they are. In the old days, you might race about gathering spider webs to plug things up, an old folk remedy believed to stop the bleeding. Lucky for you, there are better ways now to both prevent and treat this pesky problem.

Your nose is rich in blood vessels that help warm and moisten the air you breathe in. They lie close to the surface of your nasal passages, making them easier to injure. Most nosebleeds happen in the front of the nose (anterior) and stop quickly, but when they occur in the back of your nose (posterior), they can cause heavy bleeding and be much more serious. If you feel blood draining down the back of your throat, see a doctor – you probably have a posterior nosebleed, which is more common in older adults.

Older adults tend to suffer more severe nosebleeds, too, thanks to atherosclerosis, high blood pressure, and blood-thinning drugs. Blood vessels hardened from atherosclerosis can't contract to slow a nosebleed the way healthy vessels can, so the bleeding tends to last longer, especially if you also have high blood pressure. Plus, blood-thinning drugs like warfarin (Coumadin), dipyridamole (Persantine), aspirin, ibuprofen, and other nonsteroidal anti-inflammatory drugs (NSAIDs) make it harder for your blood to clot.

There are a couple of easy things you can do to help prevent nosebleeds.

- Sneeze with your mouth open.
- Stop smoking. This bad habit dries out and irritates your nasal passages, setting the stage for nosebleeds.
- Clip your nails. Nose picking is one of the most common causes of nosebleeds. If you're going to do it, at least keep your fingernails short so you don't scratch your nasal passages.

First aid for bloody noses

Nosebleeds are no fun, but you can treat almost all of them at home. Stay calm and follow this first-aid advice to staunch the flow and prevent future nosebleeds.

- Sit down and lean forward so the blood drains out your nostrils and not down the back of your throat. Spit out any blood you feel in your throat – don't swallow it.
- While leaning forward, pinch your nose between the hard bridge and the soft tip, and apply pressure until it stops bleeding. Check it after five minutes. If your nose is still bleeding, pinch it for another 10 minutes without letting go.
- Lay a cold compress or ice pack across the bridge of your nose. You can also hold a piece of ice against the roof of your mouth to control bleeding.
- Spray two squirts of a nasal spray with oxymetazoline, like Afrin, in each bleeding nostril, then pinch them closed again. This medicine constricts the blood vessels inside your nose. You can also spray it on a small cotton ball and insert it into your nostril for 10 to 15 minutes.

Head to your doctor's office or an emergency room if the bleeding hasn't stopped after 15 minutes, or if it started because of an accident or injury. Get checked out if you have frequent nosebleeds, since this can signal an underlying health problem such as a nasal tumor or blood clotting disorder.

Once the bleeding stops, be extra careful not to start it again. Don't bend over, and hold off blowing your nose and taking aspirin, ibuprofen, or other nonsteroidal anti-inflammatory drugs (NSAIDs) for several days. Rest for a full 24 hours afterward, and avoid strenuous exercise, heavy lifting, and straining during bowel movements for a week. You can apply a triple antibiotic ointment inside your nostril for a week after the bleeding.

No-nonsense nose care

Keep the inside of your nose nice and moist and you can thumb your nose at nosebleeds. Start by drinking plenty of water and juices throughout the day to prevent dehydration, and then follow up with this advice.

Steam the air. Run a humidifier in your bedroom at night to prevent your nostrils from drying out. Be sure to clean the machine regularly, according to the instructions.

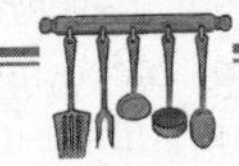

Why spend money on saline sprays when you can make your own at home and be sure of its freshness? Dissolve 1/2 teaspoon of table salt in 1 cup of warm water, then pour the mixture into a small spray bottle or a rubber bulb syringe. If this saline spray makes your nose burn, try using less salt next time.

Spray on relief. Squirt some saline nasal spray into each nostril to keep your nose moist even in the driest weather. Spray toward the septum, the wall in the middle of your nose that separates your nostrils. It's the most prone to drying out and bleeding.

Smear on some jelly. Dab a little petroleum jelly on the septum just inside each nostril to keep nasal passages lubricated. Some people react badly to long-term use of this remedy, so if you become congested or stuffed up, stop using it and see your doctor.

Osteoarthritis

Smart ways to ease symptoms

Old-time treatments for arthritis are as common as dew in Dixie – and some of them really work. Sleeping in a sleeping bag can keep your joints warm at night so you wake up with fewer aches. Bee venom might also help nip the pain of an achy joint. And if wrapping a cabbage leaf around your swollen knee works, why not try it?

Osteoarthritis (OA), the most common form of arthritis, occurs more frequently with age. Many health experts think it's caused by joint injury and a family tendency for the disease.

Pain and swelling in your joints, especially your knees, hips, feet, spine, and fingers, occur when cartilage breaks down over time. With less cartilage left to cushion a joint, the bones become damaged and react by forming spurs or knobs. Pockets of fluid can form around the joints, causing even more pain.

Although there is no cure for OA at present, these tips can help you feel well, stay active, and live longer – without dangerous drugs.

- Get some exercise every day to strengthen and loosen up your stiff joints.
- Maintain a healthy weight to reduce stress on joints.
- Make wise food choices. What you eat can affect your pain and inflammation.
- Try hot and cold therapy. You can use ice packs or heating pads – or even try alternating them to see what works best for you.

- Use adaptive tools whenever you need them. Whether you purchase items made especially for people with arthritis in their hands or simply add tape or cushioning to the handles of your tools, you can make any job easier with the right equipment.

Find out what works best in your life to keep a handle on OA, and you can go from feeling stiff as a poker to right as rain.

Spice up your life to relieve pain

You can find relief for your arthritis pain hiding in your spice rack. Turmeric, a spice found in curry powder, can help you avoid the dangerous side effects of many pain relievers. It fights inflammation and blocks the pain of both OA and rheumatoid arthritis.

Turmeric's main ingredient, curcumin, behaves like COX-2 inhibitor drugs, such as celecoxib (Celebrex). These drugs stop pain and swelling by blocking a natural enzyme called cyclooxygenase-2 (COX-2) that triggers inflammation.

You can get turmeric in your diet by eating spicy Indian curry. If you're not wild about spicy food, try turmeric supplements. Experts recommend taking 400 to 1,000 milligrams three times a day. However, some people should avoid turmeric. It can enhance the effects of blood-thinning medications, like aspirin and warfarin. It's also not recommended if you have gallstones.

Fabulous fats soothe aches

You can banish arthritis pain by choosing healthy fats. Fish oil and olive oil can help keep your joints in tip-top shape. At the same time, cut back on saturated fats and omega-6 fats, which can trigger inflammation. Saturated fats are lurking in meat, egg yolks, whole milk, ice cream, butter, and cheese, as well as palm oil and hydrogenated vegetable shortenings. Vegetable oils, like corn, safflower, soybean, and cottonseed, are high in omega-6 fats.

Fish oil. The omega-3 fatty acids in fish oil may battle both rheumatoid arthritis and osteoarthritis. Omega-3 fatty acids fight inflammation, the process that damages joints and causes pain and swelling. Recent studies show that people with OA can reduce their pain and slow cartilage damage by getting more omega-3 fatty acids.

Many health experts recommend eating at least two servings of fish, such as salmon, catfish, shrimp, herring, or canned light tuna, every week. Avoid swordfish, shark, tilefish, and king mackerel because they can contain dangerous amounts of mercury, pesticides, or other toxins. If you choose fish oil supplements, talk with your doctor to find out what dosage is right for you.

Olive oil. Olive oil, an important part of a Mediterranean diet, is a great source of monounsaturated fatty acids. These fatty acids work like omega-3s by helping to reduce joint inflammation. The Mediterranean diet also includes lots of vegetables, fruits, legumes, and grains, along with plenty of fish and small amounts of dairy products and meat.

Recently, scientists made an amazing discovery – the substance that makes extra-virgin olive oil so tangy, oleocanthal, is similar to the anti-inflammatory compound in ibuprofen.

Exercise loosens up stiff joints

You might not feel like exercising if your joints hurt, but staying active keeps your joints, and the rest of your body, healthy. For the greatest benefits, exercise regularly and include these three basic types of exercise – stretching or range-of-motion exercises; strengthening exercises, like lifting weights; and aerobics or endurance training, like walking, swimming, or another activity that gets your heart pumping. People with OA should avoid jarring exercises, such as jogging or playing racquetball.

Tai chi, an ancient Chinese form of movement, has special benefits for people with OA. This low-impact exercise can help in several ways.

MythBuster: Can copper reduce pain?

Save your money if you're thinking about buying a copper bracelet. Although promoters of these bracelets say they relieve arthritis symptoms by balancing the body's "energy force," researchers say they don't work. They tested the theory that ionized copper or zinc worn next to the body might cut joint or muscle pain. They gave one group of people ionized bracelets and another group fake "healing" bracelets. Both groups reported the same amount of pain relief during the 28-day study. The researchers attributed it to the placebo effect.

- relieves aches and pains
- improves balance
- boosts strength, endurance, and flexibility without putting too much stress on your joints

In one recent study, older people with arthritis who practiced tai chi for 10 weeks had less pain than a control group who didn't try this gentle exercise.

Another great benefit of tai chi and other forms of exercise is they keep your heart healthy and help you reduce body fat. That's important if you have OA, since carrying extra weight puts added stress on your painful joints. In fact, studies show that overweight people who lose just 5 pounds put 20 pounds less stress on their knees.

2 popular supplements: look before you leap

Glucosamine and chondroitin sulfate are popular do-it-yourself remedies for OA. Most glucosamine supplements are made from shellfish. Chondroitin comes from animal cartilage. Because the two are components of normal cartilage, many people think they can protect and rebuild the cartilage in your joints, reducing the pain of OA.

However, a recent, long-term study found they might not work for everyone. The Glucosamine/chondroitin Arthritis Intervention Trial (GAIT) followed 1,600 people with OA of the knee, comparing the use of glucosamine, chondroitin sulfate, glucosamine and chondroitin sulfate together, the drug celecoxib (Celebrex), and a sugar pill or placebo. The study, which lasted for six months, had mixed results.

For people with mild to moderate OA, glucosamine and chondroitin sulfate didn't work any better than a placebo. People with more severe arthritis, however, did benefit from the supplement combination.

Many doctors recommend trying the supplements for three months to see if they work. Check with your doctor before taking glucosamine if you are allergic to shellfish or are taking a blood thinner. And keep this mind – not all brands contain enough of the active ingredients to work well, and some don't even contain the amount listed on the label. ConsumerLab.com is an organization that

Help for weary knees

High-heeled shoes are hard on your feet – and your knees. Whether you like pointy stiletto heels or more stable wide heels, shoes with height, especially more than 2 inches, put extra pressure on your knees, which can lead to osteoarthritis over time. Surprisingly, studies show wearing wide heels is worse for your knees. Since these shoes are more comfortable, women tend to wear them longer. What's your best bet if you have OA in your knees? Wear flat shoes, or shoes with heels no higher than 2 inches, and add special wedge insoles to reduce joint stress.

tests and analyzes supplements and publishes their evaluations. For the results, go to *www.consumerlab.com* and choose "Select a review."

SAM-e battles pain and depression

SAM-e, short for S-adenosyl-methionine, is a powerful supplement used to treat arthritis and depression. Discovered in Italy in 1952 and used in Europe for many years, it's finally gaining popularity in the United States.

Your body's cells naturally make SAM-e, but they make less and less as you age. SAM-e protects your joints by helping repair cartilage, but researchers say it also fights OA pain just as well as nonsteroidal anti-inflammatory drugs (NSAIDs), like ibuprofen and naproxen – without stomach upset. SAM-e also regulates hormones and substances that transmit nerve impulses, which affect your mood.

If you want to try SAM-e supplements for your arthritis pain, some doctors recommend taking 800 milligrams (mg) a day divided into two doses. After two weeks, if you see an improvement in pain, they suggest reducing the dosage to 400 mg twice a day.

You may want to add folic acid and vitamin B12 supplements along with SAM-e because they help your body use it more effectively. Let your doctor know you are trying SAM-e, especially if you are depressed, have a mood disorder, or are taking other medication.

Rub on powerful relief

Taking a pill isn't your only choice for relieving achy joints. Arthritis pain relief is available in creams you apply to your skin. You can buy them over the counter at your favorite drugstore or discount department store. Here are two ingredients to look for.

Capsaicin. This is what makes hot peppers hot. When you rub capsaicin cream on your skin, it reduces the amount of substance P, a chemical in your body that transmits pain impulses to your brain and promotes joint inflammation. Massage capsaicin cream into the affected areas three or four times a day. If you're applying it to your hands, don't wash your hands for at least 30 minutes.

Menthol. Another proven treatment is a cream containing cetylated fatty acids, which relieve pain and improve mobility in people with knee osteoarthritis. However, in a recent study, adding menthol to the cream made it even more effective. The study participants, who suffered with OA of the knees, wrists, and elbows, had significantly less pain and greater mobility. They applied the cream twice a day for a week.

Bloodsuckers to the rescue

Leeches have been used in medicine throughout history. Although today's health professionals tend to shun these blood-sucking critters, they might hold the key to pain relief. Amazingly, leech saliva contains powerful anti-inflammatory substances that can cut pain and inflammation in people with knee osteoarthritis.

In one study, the participants undergoing leech therapy experienced a significant reduction in pain starting on the third day. More importantly, their symptoms improved for three months with just one application of leeches. Stay tuned – researchers hope to develop a pain reliever containing the anti-inflammatory substances found in leech saliva.

Osteoporosis

Stand tall with stronger bones

In the Disney movie *Snow White*, the wicked stepmother disguises herself as an elderly woman. She even adopts a stooped posture. People once thought a shrunken, stooped posture was a natural part of aging, but the real culprit is usually osteoporosis. Here's what happens to your bones.

Your skeleton constantly rebuilds itself. First, cells called osteoclasts clean out between 10 and 30 percent of old bone each year. Then cells called osteoblasts form new bone. They make it from the collagen your body produces and the phosphorus and calcium you get from food. Up until age 30, you create more bone than you lose. But as you age, you lose bone faster than you make it. Women lose the most during the first few years after menopause, but bone loss also affects men.

This happens without any symptoms or early warning signs. As osteoclasts gradually remove old bone, your bone density is reduced, meaning your bones become weaker and less solid. Little fractures in your spine may gradually reduce your height and make your posture stooped. Or you may discover you have osteoporosis when you suddenly fracture your hip or wrist.

Fortunately, you can start winning your "Battle of the Bones" today. Take up walking, gardening, or other weight-bearing exercises to help preserve bone. Ask your doctor if you should have a bone mineral density scan. Experts especially recommend a scan if you are over age 65 or if you're a woman past menopause who has had a bone fracture. And for the most amazing results, try the following remedies, too.

Good fats battle brittle bones

Here's good news for your bones. New research suggests omega-3 fats may persuade osteoclasts to remove less bone. That could put you one step closer to dodging a disabling hip fracture.

To get extra bang from these good fats, replace some weekly servings of meat and eggs with dishes that contain flaxseeds, flaxseed oil, walnuts, or oily fish like herring. You'll not only add omega-3 fats, but you'll also reduce the bone-sapping saturated fats and omega-6 fats in your diet. That's good news because too much saturated fat may lower bone density in men under age 50. What's more, most people eat too many omega-6 fats and too few omega-3s. Reversing this trend could help you beef up your bone density.

Sunshine vitamin revs up calcium

Vitamin D might help you absorb up to 65 percent more bone-saving calcium from foods and supplements, a new study claims. Although you need 1,200 milligrams (mg) of calcium daily if you're over age 50 to make and maintain bone, the average American only gets 600 mg from food.

To add more calcium, eat low-fat dairy foods, kale, turnip greens, and broccoli – along with calcium-fortified items like orange juice,

Sweet treats cheat your bones

Refined sugar may be white, but it has a dark side. It reduces the amount of calcium in your bones. Try substituting your favorite fruits for desserts, packaged snacks, and candy.

cereal, and oatmeal. Also, ask your doctor whether you need calcium supplements. If you do, try Tums or look for a supplement with the United States Pharmacopeia (USP) symbol on it. Other supplements may contain dangerous amounts of lead.

To take in more vitamin D, eat fish like tuna and salmon twice a week and enjoy fortified foods like milk and cereals. If you choose a nonfat source of vitamin D, eat a little fat with it to help you absorb this bone friendly vitamin. Your body also manufactures vitamin D when you are exposed to sunlight.

Ask your doctor whether you need extra vitamin D from a supplement to help fight osteoporosis. Many experts think the minimum recommended amount isn't enough, especially during winter when bone loss is more likely.

Tea builds a stronger skeleton

Drinking colas, both diet and regular, is linked to low bone density, a recent study shows. But if you drink tea instead of cola, you could do more than just slow your bone loss. Studies from Britain and China suggest that drinking green or black tea at least once a week means better bone density. Tea is a good source of fluoride. Fluoride not only helps your teeth, it can stimulate bone growth. What's more, tea also contains bone friendly antioxidants to help strengthen your bones. But choose decaffeinated tea because caffeine may play a role in bone loss.

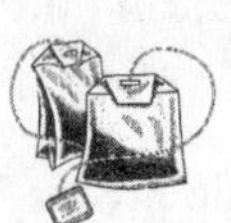

Just remember – fluoride needs calcium to help build strong bones. So drink tea, get plenty of calcium, and talk to your doctor about the latest news on fluoride and how you can get the right amount.

Zinc: manly defense for sturdy bones

Men who don't get enough zinc have lower bone density, researchers say. Although osteoporosis is considered a woman's disease, it affects as many as two out of every 10 men over age 70. Fortunately, eating more foods rich in zinc may help both men and women. Zinc not only helps vitamin D defend your bones, but this mineral also plays an important role in rebuilding bone. Ask your doctor about this bone-smart mineral at your next appointment. For now, add extra zinc by eating shellfish, red meat, barley, chickpeas, lentils, oat bran, and black beans.

DASH plan sends bone robbers packing

You may think the DASH eating plan only helps lower high blood pressure, but this clever little plan also fills your meals with bone-building nutrients. Here's what you'll reap from the DASH eating plan.

- Magnesium. This mineral helps you absorb calcium from food and reinforces new bone so it's strong instead of brittle. Get magnesium from foods like almonds, walnuts, spinach, beet greens, rye, and buckwheat.

- Vitamin K. You'll keep more bone, hang on to more calcium, and lower your risk of disabling hip fractures with vitamin K. Collard greens, romaine lettuce, asparagus, broccoli, cabbage, and other green leafy vegetables contain vitamin K. But don't load up on vitamin K if you take blood-thinning drugs, like warfarin. Talk to your doctor first.

- Vitamin C. The DASH plan is rich in the vitamin C your body needs to make collagen, one of the key ingredients in bone. Bell peppers, oranges, orange juice, cranberry juice cocktail, and broccoli are all "high C" foods.

- Potassium. Not only will this mineral help you absorb calcium, it may also prevent conditions that pull calcium out of your bones. Get extra potassium from potatoes, bananas, raisins, yogurt, tomatoes, carrots, and celery. Potassium also helps prevent the calcium and bone loss eating too much salt causes.

You should also plan to eat more veggies, fruits, and whole grains daily. And don't forget to trade saturated fats for calcium-rich nonfat or low-fat dairy products or occasional servings of oily fish, like salmon. For more information about the DASH eating plan, see the *High blood pressure* chapter.

Easy calcium for milk haters

A beef bone could help you build more bone. Just add a beef bone to a long-cooking vegetable soup recipe. The beef bone will add calcium to the soup even if there's not a drop of milk in sight. Just don't forget to remove the bone once the cooking is done.

Dynamic duo protects fragile hips

It's not your Ps and Qs you have to watch, it's your As and Bs. These vitamins can make a big difference to your bones.

Vitamin A can be a challenge – get too much or too little and you'll raise your risk of hip fractures. Even worse, the form of vitamin A called retinol, which is stored in your body fat and liver, can reach toxic levels and weaken your bones. Be careful about taking vitamin A supplements, as well as eating too many fortified foods or animal foods. Fortunately, foods like sweet potatoes, apricots, and carrots are rich in beta carotene, a nutrient your body converts into safe amounts of vitamin A.

B vitamins help you keep strong bones, too. For example, people who develop hip fractures are usually short on vitamin B6. Doctors think vitamin K can't do its part in protecting your bones without help from vitamin B6. So eat plenty of foods rich in B6, like fortified cereals, enriched rice, tuna, and chickpeas. But that's not all.

Your bone building cells need vitamin B12 to do their jobs. People who don't get enough of this key vitamin are more likely to have osteoporosis. What's more, deficiencies in B6 and B12 may also raise your level of homocysteine. More homocysteine means more danger of osteoporosis. Get more vitamin B6 and add B12-rich foods like shellfish, clam chowder, and fortified cereals.

POISON IVY

Don't let vicious vine get under your skin

As that old song goes, "You can look but you better not touch." This catchy 1950s tune by The Coasters, "Poison Ivy," could have been about a dangerous girl or the irritating plant. If you're among the majority of people who get an itchy rash from the plant's sap, you know the rest of the song – "You're gonna need an ocean of calamine lotion."

Urushiol, a chemical found in the oily sap of poison ivy, poison sumac, and poison oak, is what causes your skin to blister and itch. Like other allergic reactions, you probably won't get a rash the first time you meet with urushiol. But your immune system creates special white blood cells to counter future attacks. Next time you come in contact with urushiol, you'll probably get a rash within a couple of days.

Quick action after you touch poison ivy can keep the damage in check.

- Use rubbing alcohol to remove the sap from your skin. If you can get it off within 10 minutes, you may keep it from entering your skin. The alcohol removes your skin's protective oils, however, so steer clear of problem plants.
- Wash with lots of water. Don't use soap at this point, since it could spread the sap. Later, you'll need to take a shower with soap.
- Clean off your clothes, tools, and anything else contaminated with the sap using rubbing alcohol and water. Protect your hands during this step with disposable gloves.

You can cross your fingers and hope you don't get poison ivy again, or you can plan ahead before you go out gardening, hiking, or just enjoying nature. The old saying, "Leaves of three, let it be," is true for only some plants with urushiol, but it's a start. Learn to spot the most common types in your area.

Wear long sleeves, long pants, and socks if you expect trouble. Some people swear by Ivy Block, a lotion you apply before you venture into the great outdoors. It forms a protective barrier on your skin so urushiol can't penetrate. In a pinch, you can spray your arms and legs with deodorant to get a similar effect. If you burn leaves, be sure there's no poison ivy in the pile. You can get urushiol in your lungs from particles in the air.

When it comes to poison ivy, there's good news and bad news. The good news is even without treatment a rash should clear up within three weeks. The bad news is researchers expect the rising level of carbon dioxide in the earth's atmosphere will encourage poison ivy to grow faster and produce even more urushiol. Like the song says, "She'll really do you in if you let her under your skin."

Hot and cold stop the itching fast

Itching from a poison ivy rash sends most people searching for relief. You may be able to fool your itchy skin using cold or heat.

MythBuster: Is poison ivy contagious?

You can get a poison ivy rash after touching urushiol, a chemical in the plant's oily sap. If you touch poison ivy leaves – or anything that came in contact with the plant – you can develop a rash. That means pet fur, clothing, gardening tools, or even another person. You can also spread the oil from one part of your body to another if you don't wash it off completely. But after a rash develops, don't worry about spreading it. The weeping blisters don't cause it to spread.

Cooling your rash is one quick, cheap way to block the itch. If there's no blister, hold an ice cube to the rash for about a minute. You can also try a cold compress for a similar effect. Make it with cold whole milk for added benefits. The milk's fat helps dry up the rash and calm the itch. Also, the lactic acid in milk is a mild alpha hydroxy acid, which can help remove dead skin cells and allow new skin cells to replace them. Place the milk compress on your rash for about 10 minutes. If necessary, repeat every hour until your skin feels better. Or try a cool compress with Burow's solution, available at most drugstores.

Some people find itch relief from heat rather than cold. You can try taking hot showers, but don't use water so hot you burn your skin. Other people like to aim a hair dryer at their stubborn poison ivy rash to block the itch – just don't get too close to your skin.

3 simple secrets for itch relief

A poison ivy reaction causes severe itching, redness, and swelling, often with weeping blisters. Take care of the rash by washing with mild soap and water and covering the weeping blisters with gauze.

Some experts say over-the-counter hydrocortisone cream is not strong enough for poison ivy itching. Instead, they suggest these remedies. If one remedy doesn't work, try another.

- Take a colloidal oatmeal bath. This finely ground oatmeal cleans your skin and leaves a protective film after it dries. Make your own by grinding about 1 cup dry oatmeal in a food processor or blender until it's a fine powder.
- Rub on the old standby, calamine lotion. It creates a film to make your skin less sensitive.
- Apply a baking soda paste to dry the blisters and relieve the pain and itch. Use one part water to three parts baking soda.

Scratching your blisters can cause them to become infected by bacteria from your fingernails. See a doctor if your rash gets worse or affects your face or large areas of your body.

PROSTATE HEALTH

Natural ways to get back to normal

Being a man has benefits, but having a prostate probably isn't one of them. The majority of men deal with prostate problems at some point in their life. Because of this organ's location, that often means dealing with urinary and sexual problems, too.

Your prostate is a gland roughly the size and shape of a crab apple, but with the apple core removed. A tube called the urethra carries urine from your bladder to your penis and outside your body. On the way there, it runs through the "hollow core" of your prostate gland. The prostate makes prostatic fluid, which it squeezes into the urethra during sex. There, it mixes with sperm to create semen. For such a small organ, a lot can go wrong. Fortunately, doctors know more than ever about preventing and treating such problems.

Watch for an enlarged prostate. In your mid-40s, the prostate gland begins to grow, a condition called benign prostatic hyperplasia (BPH). It's one of the most common ailments you face as a man. About half of all men ages 51 to 60 have enlarged prostates, as do nine in 10 men over age 80.

This overgrowth can put pressure on your urethra, interfering with the flow of urine. Your bladder has to work harder to push urine out, which in turn causes your bladder walls to thicken, so it holds less urine. You may feel the urge to urinate more often as well as have trouble starting or a weak stream. Your bladder may not empty all the way after a while, raising your risk of bladder and kidney infections. While BPH may be aggravating, it's not life threatening, nor does it increase your risk of prostate cancer. In fact, doctors only recommend treating it if the symptoms become bothersome or you get frequent urinary tract infections.

Deal with prostatitis. This inflammation of the prostate strikes almost half of all men, usually in their early 40s. You can get one of two types – bacterial and nonbacterial. Ninety-five percent of men have nonbacterial prostatitis. Doctors don't know for sure what causes it, but some suspect it is an autoimmune disorder where your immune system mistakenly attacks healthy prostate tissue.

Short-term (acute) bacterial infections tend to cause symptoms a lot like the flu – sudden fever, chills, body aches, and nausea along with pain in the pelvis or genital area, painful urination, urgency, and needing to go frequently. Chronic bacterial infections feel similar but with milder symptoms that come and go. The nonbacterial form causes the same urinary burning, urgency, and frequency along with pain in your lower back, lower abdomen, and genital area.

Get checked for prostate cancer. It's the second most common cause of cancer deaths after lung cancer. Still, while 16 out of 100 men will get prostate cancer, only three will die from it, and the death rate continues to drop. You are most likely to get this disease

Hidden risks of herbal remedies

Natural remedies that claim to boost your sex life or treat prostate problems aren't always what they're cracked up to be. Investigators have found "natural" herbal products, especially from China and Asia, laced with prescription drugs such as steroids and contaminated with toxic metals. Other products don't even contain the herbs they claim.

The Food and Drug Administration (FDA) does not regulate herbs, vitamins, and other supplements, so you never really know what you're getting. Be wary when buying them, especially those that claim to enhance your libido, treat erectile dysfunction, or improve your sex life.

if you are between the ages of 65 and 70, black, and have a brother or father who also had it.

The signs of prostate cancer closely mimic those of BPH – trouble urinating, erectile dysfunction, and the urgent need to urinate and go more often – but they usually strike suddenly. If you develop these symptoms, don't assume you have an enlarged prostate. See your doctor so he can rule out prostate cancer.

Doctors usually treat prostate problems with drugs and surgery, both of which can lead to temporary impotence. Luckily, you can take natural steps to manage symptoms and side effects and prevent prostate disorders in the first place.

Herbal healing for enlarged prostate

You may not feel lucky if you have an enlarged prostate (benign prostatic hyperplasia), but in one way, you are. More natural supplements treat this condition with some success than almost any other disease. These three supplements look particularly promising. As always, tell your doctor if you decide to take any supplement so he can avoid prescribing medications that interact with it.

Saw palmetto. Studies testing a high-quality saw palmetto supplement called Permixon have by and large found it helps symptoms of benign prostatic hyperplasia (BPH) about as well as alpha-blockers such as finasteride (Proscar), often prescribed for BPH. However, a new, larger clinical trial found saw palmetto did not improve urine flow, prostate size, bladder emptying, or quality of life in men with enlarged prostates. The debate continues.

Still, it may be worth trying, especially since it doesn't cause erectile dysfunction the way finasteride can. Shop for supplements that contain 85 percent fatty acids and 0.2 percent sterols. If your symptoms don't improve after a month, stop taking it.

African pygeum. South African tribes have long used African pygeum, the bark of the African plum tree, to treat urinary problems.

Now, 17 studies involving almost 1,000 men suggest it improves the nighttime urination, bladder emptying, and urinary frequency of BPH. Pygeum seems to put a damper on prostate inflammation and squash the overgrowth of prostate cells.

In fact, the evidence supporting pygeum is about as strong as that behind saw palmetto. The biggest difference – saw palmetto costs much less, thanks to the scarcity of the African plum tree. If you decide to try it, buy a supplement with 14 percent triterpenes and 0.5 percent n-docosanol, and take 50 milligrams (mg) twice a day.

Beta-sitosterol. Plants naturally contain cholesterol-like compounds called sitosterols. A special mixture of these compounds, beta-sitosterol, may treat enlarged prostates, although researchers don't fully understand why. Look for a supplement standardized to contain 0.2 mg of beta-sitosterol glucosides, and take 20 mg three times daily. Be sure to buy beta-sitosterol supplements formulated specifically for BPH. Some are sold to lower cholesterol, and they have very different dosage instructions.

5 steps to leak-free living

Living with an enlarged prostate can make you feel tied to the closest bathroom, what with the sudden, frequent urge to urinate and the leaky bladder that goes with it. Cut the bonds between you and the bathroom with five simple steps.

- Stop drinking fluids after 7 p.m. to cut down nighttime trips to the bathroom, and avoid drinking too much fluid in one sitting.
- Keep alcohol to a minimum. Drinking heavily can irritate your lower urinary tract.
- Take decongestants and antihistamines sparingly. They can worsen urinary symptoms and keep your bladder from emptying completely.
- Stay warm as much as possible. The cold causes your prostate to squeeze the urethra harder, making urinary symptoms worse.

- Discuss your diuretics with your doctor. These drugs make you urinate more often, a problem if you have BPH. Your doctor may be able to switch your prescription or lower the dosage. Do not stop taking them without his permission.

Easy exercise ends impotence, incontinence

Men who undergo surgery for an enlarged prostate or prostate cancer can face another hurdle afterward – the loss of bladder control and erections. Luckily, one easy exercise can help treat everything from post-surgery incontinence and impotence to erectile dysfunction caused by poor circulation.

Kegel exercises strengthen the muscles of your pelvic floor that support your bladder, control urination, and close the anal sphincter. After undergoing radical prostatectomy, 68 percent of men who did Kegels for three months conquered their urinary incontinence, compared to only 37 percent of men who did not do them.

Cancer-kicking two-step

Age and genetics play a pretty big role in developing prostate cancer, but you can take two major steps to drastically drop that risk.

- **Exercise more.** Men over the age of 65 who get a vigorous workout three hours a week can slash their risk of advanced prostate cancer nearly 70 percent. The extra physical activity may affect the hormones that drive cancer growth.
- **Lose weight.** Obese men tend to develop higher-grade prostate cancer and are more likely to see it return after surgery. Experts think the extra fat in your body raises blood levels of certain hormones that feed the cancer's growth.

Figuring out where these muscles are is probably the hardest part. Begin by practicing in the bathroom while urinating. Squeeze the muscles that stop or slow the flow of urine. Keep squeezing for three seconds, let go for three seconds, then squeeze again. Start out doing the exercise 15 times, three times a day, and gradually add more.

Once you learn where and what to squeeze, don't continue doing Kegels while urinating. You may eventually weaken the muscles. Instead, do each set in a different position – one standing, one sitting, and one lying down. You may have to exercise regularly for several months to see significant improvement, so don't give up. And discuss your problems with your doctor. He can follow your progress and offer advice to help you get back to normal.

Pomegranates crush prostate cancer

When Pluto kidnapped Persephone to make her his wife in Greek myth, she refused to eat or drink anything in the Underworld, for fear she would be trapped there forever. Like Eve with the apple, though, Persephone finally gave in to the temptation of a delicious red fruit – the pomegranate.

Had she known how healthy it is, she might have given in sooner. Far from dooming you, the juice from this exotic fruit can make prostate cancer cells self-destruct, slow the growth of the disease, and possibly keep it from spreading. In one recent study, a daily 8-ounce drink of pure pomegranate juice slowed prostate cancer progression for 4½ years in men who already had the disease. Scientists don't know yet whether it can prevent this cancer in healthy men, but, in the meantime, grab a glass and enjoy.

Special diet slashes cancer risk

Certain foods can help both prevent prostate cancer and slow its progression once you have it, while eating others raises your risk of this deadly disease. Try this anti-cancer diet on for size.

Trim the fat. In general, eating lots of fatty food seems to raise your risk of prostate cancer, while low-fat diets may slow tumor growth. Animal fat from foods like meat and milk are worst. Omega-3 fats from fish, on the other hand, may protect you, since men who eat fish at least twice a week enjoy a lower risk of prostate cancer than those who don't. Why? Certain fats may boost your blood levels of androgens, hormones that encourage the growth of prostate cancer.

Give red meat a rest. It's high in saturated fat, which may partly explain why it increases your prostate cancer risk. Some studies also link high-heat cooking – grilling, broiling, and pan-frying – to a hike in cancer risk. Plus, overcooking meat creates compounds called heterocyclic amines. Research links these substances to cancerous changes throughout the body, especially the prostate.

Eat your vegetables. Mom knew what she was talking about. Men who ate an average of four or more vegetable servings daily in a recent study dropped their prostate cancer risk 35 percent compared to eating two servings a day.

Cabbage, broccoli, cauliflower, watercress, and other cruciferous veggies boast even more benefits. Eating just three or more servings weekly gave men a 41 percent lower risk than eating them less than once a week. These special veggies contain compounds that seem to slow the development of cancer, so serve up a side, and dig in.

Cooked tomato products like tomato sauce pack more lycopene than raw tomatoes. Cooking tomatoes in olive oil will double the lycopene you absorb.

Tomatoes also lend lots of protection. They're loaded with lycopene, a powerful plant chemical that helps neutralize dangerous compounds in your body known as free radicals.

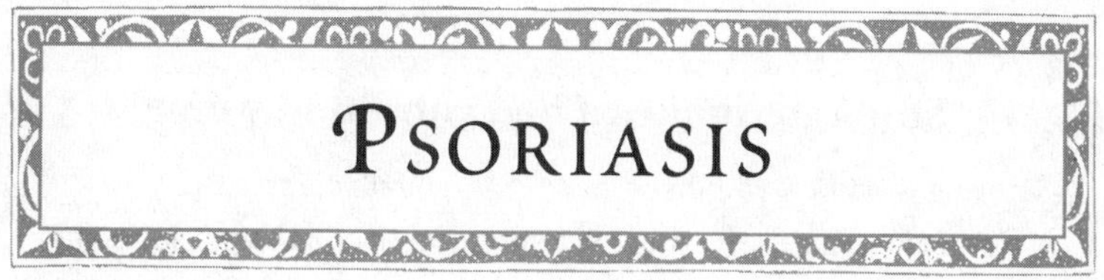

Psoriasis

Simple solutions provide hope

It's as old as the hills and, like beauty, appears to be only skin deep. But psoriasis is nothing to scoff at. People with this common condition deal with stares and questions from others, flare-ups that come from out of the blue, occasional joint problems, and expensive and time-consuming treatments – all lasting a lifetime.

Psoriasis is marked by itchy red skin patches covered by scaly flakes. Some people have a family tendency for the problem, but it's not all about genetics. Psoriasis occurs when the immune system gets out of whack and certain white blood cells gang up against other body cells. This brings on inflammation and causes keratinocytes – skin cells – to reproduce much faster than normal. The most common form, plaque psoriasis, tends to appear on your elbows, knees, and lower back, but it can also show up on your scalp, palms, soles, groin, and legs. Other forms of psoriasis attack your joints or nails.

Stress, illness, depression, hormones, and some drugs can trigger a psoriasis flare-up. Cold, dry weather can make it worse, while balmy summer conditions can clear it up. Sunlight or treatment with artificial ultraviolet (UV) light helps by destroying the skin cells that reproduce too quickly. Prescription creams like corticosteroids, salicylic acid, or those made from vitamin D3 (calcipotriene) or vitamin A (tazarotene) work well for mild to moderate psoriasis.

People with severe psoriasis may need more powerful drugs that treat the whole body – pills or shots like methotrexate, acitretin, or cyclosporine. New biologics, including alefacept and etanercept, target

Smoking makes a bad condition worse

Smoking is bad for your heart and lungs, and it's no treat for your skin, either. Smokers are more likely to have skin problems, including psoriasis, skin cancer, wrinkling, and poor wound healing. In fact, a study in Italy found that people with psoriasis who are heavy smokers often have a worse form of the disease. Those who smoke more than one pack of cigarettes a day are twice as likely to have serious symptoms as those who smoke less than half a pack a day. More years spent smoking also leads to worse flare-ups.

certain immune system cells to keep them from turning against your own body. But many of these drugs have serious side effects, including liver and kidney damage, osteoporosis, skin cancer, and high blood pressure.

People have been dealing with psoriasis for nearly 3,000 years, so they've come up with some ingenious remedies. Folk treatments include rubbing on salt, snail slime, and the ashes of burned animal hair. Other old-time ideas involve eating peanut butter and drinking various medicines. People are still willing to try alternative cures, such as bathing with "doctorfish" that nibble away at dead, flaky skin patches.

But experts suggest you deal with your psoriasis by getting enough rest and exercise, managing your stress, avoiding too much alcohol, and keeping your weight in check. Then try the cream or drug that battles your symptoms with the fewest side effects.

Make changes from the inside out

Psoriasis symptoms often clear up when people switch to low-calorie or vegetarian diets. To get the most benefit from altering your diet, follow this expert advice.

Favor fish oil. Eating fats with lots of omega-6 fatty acids, like red meats and corn oil, can lead to inflammation. But fats with omega-3 fatty acids, like fish oil, do just the opposite. Several clinical trials have shown that taking fish oil supplements helps improve psoriasis symptoms, including scales, redness, and itching. Talk to your doctor before you try this treatment, since you need to take a large daily dose of fish oil. You may also benefit from eating more oily fish like salmon and mackerel.

Try some turmeric. This popular Indian spice contains curcumin, a traditional remedy for inflammation. It's being tested to treat several conditions, including cancer, arthritis, cystic fibrosis, Alzheimer's disease, and psoriasis. If you don't like the taste of turmeric, a main ingredient in curry dishes, you can get it in supplements. But stay away from turmeric if you have gallbladder problems – it can cause potentially harmful contractions.

Go gluten-free. Some people with psoriasis also have an allergy to the gluten in wheat products. If that's you, then your psoriasis symptoms get worse after you eat foods with wheat, rye, barley, oats, and other grains. A study of people with gluten sensitivity found their psoriasis improved greatly after three months on a gluten-free diet.

It's not easy to eat a balanced diet while avoiding gluten since it's in so many breads, pastas, cereals, and similar foods. You also need to check labels of drugs and processed foods like ketchup, mustard, salad dressing, candy bars, and instant coffee, which may have gluten added. But by making the effort, you may get the relief you need.

Kick up the caffeine. If you take methotrexate or sulfasalazine for psoriasis, drinking coffee may help your drugs work better. A small study found people with psoriasis who drank 10 or more cups of coffee each week reported their drugs did a better job of relieving symptoms. Experts think the caffeine lowers your body's level of an immune protein that brings on inflammation.

MythBuster: Can you catch psoriasis?

Large areas of scaly skin and red patches on someone with psoriasis can be unsightly, but there's no reason to shrink away. Psoriasis is not contagious, so you can't catch it by touching someone with the disease or by handling her clothing. Doctors don't know exactly what causes psoriasis, but they think some people's immune systems overreact, encouraging the skin to make new cells way too fast. Stress, weather, and other changes can bring on a flare-up. So don't shy away from a friend with psoriasis – offer her help and support.

Rub-on remedies offer first-line defense

Many pills and shots for psoriasis have side effects, so doctors recommend you first try creams and ointments to treat your symptoms. Even some topical remedies, including corticosteroid and vitamin D3 creams, cause problems like itching, burning, and thinning of the skin. But you can get relief without a prescription from these simple choices.

Aloe vera. Gel from the leaves of this plant, best known for burn relief, also battles inflammation to clear up psoriasis symptoms. You can apply the gel straight from the plant or buy aloe vera cream. Rub it on your psoriasis patches three times a day.

Coal tar. This old remedy keeps skin cells from reproducing too quickly. Shampoos and creams with coal tar work for mild to moderate psoriasis, although they can smell bad, irritate your skin, and stain your clothes. Be careful if you have light-colored hair – coal-tar shampoo can give it an orange tint.

Oregon grape. Extract from the Oregon grape shrub looks promising as a psoriasis treatment. A study of 200 people found Reliéva, a cream made from Oregon grape extract, worked better than a placebo on psoriasis symptoms when they used it twice a day for 12 weeks. Like coal tar, Oregon grape extract cream can irritate your skin and stain your clothes. If you want to try it, you can buy Reliéva online or at a health-food store.

Cheap choices battle dryness and itch

You don't need to break open your piggy bank to buy pricy creams and lotions that fight the itchy, dry skin of psoriasis. Experts say the best inexpensive remedies are things you may already have at home.

Mix in petroleum jelly. For dry skin – no matter what the cause – petroleum jelly is a great solution that won't cause irritation. Like other emollients, it creates a barrier to keep in your body's own moisture. If your doctor prescribes a topical vitamin A drug, which can dry and irritate your skin, try blending it with petroleum jelly until you get used to the treatment.

Enjoy another use for olive oil. Rub the oil directly on your patches of psoriasis. It's a great natural moisturizer, and it won't irritate your skin like some fancy creams.

Relax in an oatmeal bath. Oatmeal is an old-time soothing remedy for itching and dryness. Try a bath with colloidal oatmeal added – whole oat grain ground up into a fine powder. You can also mix two cups oatmeal with four cups water and boil to create a paste. Be careful when you step into the tub, however, since it will be slippery.

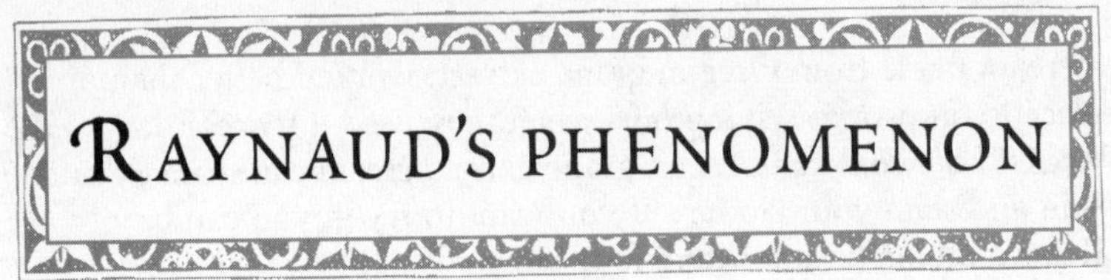

Raynaud's phenomenon

Speedy help for cold hands

"Cold hands, warm heart," is probably your motto if you suffer from Raynaud's phenomenon. This blood vessel disorder can suddenly leave your fingers and toes numb, bloodless, and blue – a frightening sight no matter how often it happens. Luckily, you can manage it yourself, typically without drugs or surgery.

Your blood vessels naturally narrow when you are out in the cold for long periods. This restricts blood flow to your hands and feet in order to keep the organs in the center of your body warm. During stressful situations, something similar happens – your body releases hormones that narrow your blood vessels.

In Raynaud's, your body overreacts to these triggers. Your response to cold happens faster and stronger than normal, and during times of stress, your blood vessels squeeze closed harder than they should. This dramatic narrowing cuts off blood flow to your fingers, toes, and, in rare cases, your nose, lips, ears, and nipples. Your fingers and other affected areas may turn white then blue and either hurt or go numb. They may tingle and turn red when your blood vessels reopen and blood returns to the area.

You can have one of two types of Raynaud's – primary, where doctors can't find a cause, or secondary, where an underlying condition like scleroderma, lupus, rheumatoid arthritis, or atherosclerosis is causing your blood vessels to narrow. Women between the ages of 15 and 40 are most likely to develop the disorder, as are people living in colder climates. Primary Raynaud's is more common, but secondary Raynaud's is usually more severe.

Most people with primary Raynaud's can control it with simple lifestyle changes. If you have secondary Raynaud's, you may also need medication or, in rare cases, surgery. Start with these steps and see if they curb your symptoms.

- Stop smoking. Nicotine narrows your arteries, restricts blood flow, and can make the temperature of your skin drop, triggering an attack.

- Cut out caffeine. It naturally constricts your blood vessels, which decreases blood flow. Aside from coffee, watch out for hidden caffeine in soda, tea, and chocolate.

- Kick back and relax. Avoid stressful situations and learn to let go of worries and handle stress in healthy ways.

- Seek treatment for underlying conditions if you suffer with secondary Raynaud's.

- Check your medicine cabinet for drugs linked to secondary Raynaud's, including ergotamines (for migraines), beta-blockers (for high blood pressure), and drugs containing pseudoephedrine (for colds and allergies). Talk to your doctor if you think medications are causing your attacks, but don't stop taking drugs prescribed by your doctor without his approval.

For most people, the symptoms are little more than annoying, but for people with severe Raynaud's, frequent attacks or prolonged blood loss can lead to sores and gangrene. See your doctor immediately if you develop sores on your fingers, toes, or other areas.

Toasty tips keep attacks at bay

Simply staying warm, dry, and hydrated can go a long way toward alleviating attacks when you have Raynaud's. Try these crafty ideas for keeping the cold away.

- Wear gloves, mittens, or oven mitts when reaching into the freezer or refrigerator and handling cold food at the supermarket.

- Bump up the thermostat at home, especially during summer when you run the air conditioner. Air conditioning can set off a Raynaud's attack.
- Dress in warm layers in air-conditioned places, like the office, church, or movie theater.
- Shop for socks made of wool, synthetic material, or a cotton blend. They keep your feet warmer and drier than 100-percent cotton socks.
- Enjoy a hot cup of decaffeinated tea or steamy bowl of soup before heading out in cold weather. Eating increases your body temperature, which helps you stay warm.
- Invest in insulated drinking glasses for cold beverages and coozies for cold cans and bottles to protect your hands.
- Wear a hat outdoors in winter and indoors in summer if air conditioning makes you freeze. Choose one that covers your ears or wear earmuffs.
- Sleep wearing socks, mittens, and a soft hat when the weather turns cold.
- Drink plenty of fluids. Dehydration can lower the amount of blood moving through your blood vessels, triggering or worsening an attack.
- Add a dash of foot powder inside shoes to keep your feet dry. Wet feet get cold easier.
- Consider buying small pouches filled with chemicals that heat up when activated. Tuck them in pockets, socks, shoes, or gloves when you are out in the cold for long periods.

3 natural alternatives offer relief

Several supplements show promise in treating primary Raynaud's phenomenon. Scientists are still researching them but say these three could help defrost your frozen fingers and toes.

Get back feeling with ginkgo. The Chinese cure-all ginkgo biloba increases circulation in your fingertips, and experts suspect it also tones up blood vessels and makes them more elastic. People with primary Raynaud's who took 120 milligrams of the herb three times a day for 10 weeks had half as many attacks as usual. Ginkgo can thin your blood, so discuss it with your doctor first. Don't use it if you take blood-thinning medications, such as warfarin (Coumadin) or aspirin.

Catch "reel" relief from fish oil. In one small trial, people with Raynaud's found daily fish oil capsules curbed their bodies' reaction to cold. Other studies suggest you need as much as 12 grams of fish oil daily to see results, a much higher dose than normal. Talk to your doctor before treating your Raynaud's with this remedy. Fish oil also thins your blood, so don't take it if you are on blood-thinning drugs. Shop for supplements certified not to contain PCBs, mercury, or other contaminants.

Beat symptoms with B3. Inositol hexaniacinate, a form of the B vitamin niacin, seems to improve Raynaud's symptoms, increase blood flow, and reduce the number of attacks. The results are promising, but

Exterminate gut bug to dodge Raynaud's

Consider being tested for the *H. pylori* bacterium, especially if you have digestive problems along with your Raynaud's symptoms. Research has linked this bad bug, famous for causing ulcers, to primary Raynaud's.

In an Italian study, an amazing 78 percent of people with primary Raynaud's also had an *H. pylori* infection. Six weeks of antibiotics killed off the infection in 30 out of 36 people. Of those, five saw their Raynaud's symptoms completely disappear, while 18 had significantly fewer and shorter attacks. The six people who still had *H. pylori* after taking antibiotics saw no improvement.

you may need to take it long term to see any benefits. You may also need to take it in high doses, as much as 4 grams a day. Doses this large can lead to liver inflammation, so avoid inositol supplements if you have liver disease, gout, a history of ulcers, or if you drink alcohol regularly. Be careful of this vitamin even if you don't have one of these conditions. You should only try it under your doctor's supervision so he can periodically check your liver function.

Kitchen spices heat up Raynaud's

Common kitchen seasonings, such as cayenne, mustard powder, and horseradish, can help keep you warm and boost circulation. They are rubefacients, substances you put on your skin that dilate blood vessels and increase circulation.

People once sprinkled cayenne inside their socks to keep their feet warm on cold nights. No research has tested these remedies specifically for Raynaud's, a blood vessel disorder marked by poor circulation in your hands and feet. However, they might help fight off the cold that triggers an attack and get your blood flowing.

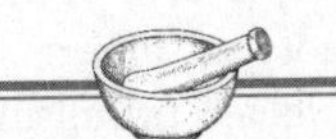

Once an attack starts, it's important to get blood flowing back into the area. Hold your arms out from your sides and whirl them around like a windmill. You can also open and close your hands into fists or shake them until the attack passes. All of these exercises help send blood back into the arteries in your hands.

Try sprinkling cayenne powder in your shoes or socks if you want to try the old folk remedy. Or soak your feet in a mustard bath by steeping one tablespoon of mustard seeds in about a quart of hot water.

Rubefacients like these can irritate sensitive skin, so test them on a small area of skin first. Don't get them in your eyes or nose, and never apply them to broken skin. Wash your hands thoroughly after handling them.

Restless Legs Syndrome

Smooth steps to soothe the fidgeting

The nighttime twitching, prickling, skin-crawling sensations deep in your legs is the stuff made of nightmares, but it's not in your head. The uncontrollable urge to move your legs, often accompanied by painful sensations in your calves, may be a sign of restless legs syndrome (RLS). This disorder afflicts about 10 percent of people and up to 35 percent of adults over age 65.

These odd feelings get worse at night, particularly when you rest. You can relieve them by moving or rubbing your legs, but as soon as you stop, the symptoms come back. Eventually, you may get these creepy sensations during the day, too, and discover that moving your legs no longer calms them.

As if RLS isn't bad enough on its own, about 80 percent of people who suffer with it also have periodic limb movement disorder (PLMD), where your legs jerk repeatedly during sleep but without waking you up as RLS does. This combination can make for especially rough nights. People with restless legs syndrome tend to be sleep-deprived and especially tired during the day, more prone to insomnia, depression, anxiety, headaches, and low sex drive.

RLS tends to run in families, but other people can develop it, too. Scientists have spotted several genetic links to the disorder. Certain medications and health problems such as anemia and renal failure can also trigger it. In these cases, treating the underlying condition, like iron deficiency, or changing your medication may make your symptoms disappear.

Changing your eating and living habits is the first line of defense against RLS, but your doctor will prescribe medication if options like these don't help.

- Steer clear of alcohol, caffeine, and cigarettes, all of which aggravate RLS.
- Cut back on stress, and talk to your doctor about learning relaxation techniques.
- Walk briskly for 30 minutes a day, and try to lift weights with your lower body three times a week. People with RLS who followed this exercise plan improved their symptoms 39 percent in only six weeks – about the same length of time it takes medication to work.

Iron out the kinks in your diet

Low iron levels are one of the main culprits behind secondary restless legs syndrome. In fact, studies have shown as many as 30

Rx for restless legs

Before you go in for expensive tests and treatments, check your medicine cabinet. These and other drugs can trigger secondary restless legs syndrome or make existing symptoms worse.

- antihistamines
- antipsychotics
- certain calcium channel blockers
- antidepressants, including fluoxetine (Prozac) and lithium (Eskalith), but not bupropion (Wellbutrin, Zyban), which may improve restless legs syndrome symptoms
- anti-nausea drugs, including metoclopramide (Reglan), prochlorperazine (Compazine), and chlorpromazine (Thorazine), but not granisetron hydrochloride (Kytril) or ondansetron hydrochloride (Zofran)

percent of people with low iron levels have RLS. A poor diet, renal failure, gastrointestinal bleeding, even giving blood too often, can lead to low levels of iron in your blood or in the fluid surrounding your brain. Either can translate into too little dopamine, a brain chemical that helps control the movements of your arms and legs.

Food has two types of iron – heme, found in seafood and meat; and non-heme, found mostly in vegetables, eggs, and dairy products. You absorb heme iron better than non-heme, but both help boost your iron levels. These tips can help you get more of this mineral from your everyday meals.

- Cook food in cast iron skillets and pans to get more iron into your meals.
- Serve up lean meat and fish. They're packed with heme iron, and they'll help you absorb non-heme iron.
- Boil, steam, or stir-fry vegetables in any kind of pot or pan to release their non-heme iron.
- Skip drinking tea, coffee, or red wine with meals. Compounds called polyphenols in these beverages keep your body from taking up the iron in food.
- Have a glass of orange juice, instead. Vitamin C helps you absorb non-heme iron. Drinking just 6 ounces of OJ with a meal can double the iron you soak up from plant foods. Add in other C-rich foods like citrus fruits, broccoli, tomatoes, and strawberries.

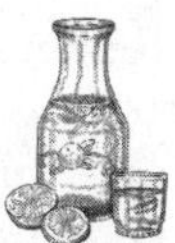

Attack RLS by increasing the iron you get from food, and talk to your doctor before you try supplements. Iron pills only help people who are truly deficient.

Relaxing bedtime habits calm jittery limbs

Non-drug therapies are the first line of treatment for RLS. Establishing a bedtime routine can help. Before you face another sleepless night, try this recipe for calming restless legs.

Slow down. Lots of exercise or stimulation, including sex, within one or two hours of bedtime can lead to a bad night of RLS. Instead, end your day with gentle stretching and a leg massage. Other people claim relief from hot, cold, or alternating hot and cold baths or compresses, although cold aggravates symptoms in some people.

Engage your brain. You've probably discovered that physical activity relieves RLS. Strangely enough, so can mental workouts. Any mind-challenging pastime that engrosses you, like painting, needlepoint, crossword puzzles, or interesting conversations take your mind off your legs when you aren't moving. Occupy yourself with an engaging pastime as you relax before bed.

Set a sleep schedule. Try to go to bed and wake up at the same time every day, even on weekends. RLS usually peaks around midnight, and some sufferers say they sleep better late in the morning. See if staying up late and sleeping in works for you.

Stop suppressing it. If your symptoms keep you awake, stop trying to ignore them. Get out of bed and do something mentally engaging to get your mind off your discomfort.

Simple ways to take back your life

Restless legs impact your days as well as your nights. They keep you awake when you need to sleep and keep you from sitting still to do the things you enjoy, like reading or watching movies. Take back your life with a few changes in your routine.

- Raise your desk or computer high enough for you to stand while you read or work. Sit on a high stool and dangle your legs while you read. Some people find this helps calm their legs.
- Grab an aisle seat during long flights or when sitting in the theater. You can stretch your legs out and fidget without disturbing others.
- Invest in a cordless phone so you can talk to friends and walk at the same time.

Rheumatoid Arthritis

Bring 'rheumatism' into the modern age

Did your grandma moan over joint pain when her "rheumatism" acted up? Did she try to ease the ache by carrying a buckeye or a potato in her pocket? She might have been relying on folk remedies to treat a condition now called rheumatoid arthritis (RA).

This painful disease occurs when your body literally turns against itself. Although experts don't completely understand why this happens, the bottom line is your immune system attacks your joints. Rogue molecules cause the cushioning cartilage to break down, and the result is throbbing, warm, swollen joints. Over time, RA even damages your bones. It's more common in women, and most often affects the joints in your hands, wrists, knees, and feet. Unlike osteoarthritis, morning stiffness from RA usually lasts more than an hour, and matching joints – like both hands or both knees – are often affected.

If you have these symptoms of early RA, see a doctor for treatment to keep it from getting worse. Research shows some people who begin drug therapy early can avoid more serious joint damage. Doctors often suggest first taking nonsteroidal anti-inflammatory drugs (NSAIDs) to battle the pain and swelling. But there are stronger drugs that can suppress your immune system or keep your cells from attacking each other. Unfortunately, all of them have side effects – some very serious.

Once RA is diagnosed, you can help your joints feel better by taking these steps.

Rest when you need it. This is especially important if more than one joint is hurting – it will help reduce inflammation. Feeling overly tired is a serious problem for some people with RA, so listen to your body.

Keep moving. When you can, get some exercise to keep joints flexible, build muscle strength, and increase your endurance and mobility. Stretching, mild strength training, dancing, swimming, and walking are all good choices. But avoid high-impact activities like running and jumping.

Eat right. Your body must have the nutrients it needs to battle inflammation and its symptoms. Doctors see a strong link between RA inflammation and heart disease, so it's important to follow a heart-healthy diet. One of the most highly recommended is the Mediterranean diet. To follow it, you should eat monounsaturated fats like olive oil; fish as a protein source; garlic; complex carbohydrates from whole grains, beans, nuts, and fresh fruits and vegetables; and wine, if you choose.

Shop for help. Try a brace or splint on your affected joint to keep it supported and correctly aligned. Think about buying a few devices or appliances that make day-to-day activities easier, like jar openers, zipper pulls, or gripping tools.

Grandma might have been right about a lot of things, but you should skip the rheumatism snake oil and try basic healthy living to keep your RA in check.

Antioxidants: colorful cure for inflammation

Eating your fruits and veggies is one way to battle RA. Several studies have shown specific foods can act in certain ways to reduce the risk of RA and soothe the inflammation that causes joint damage.

Bone up on nutritional knowledge. Oxidation is as natural as breathing. In fact, it is caused by breathing. With every breath you take, you bring life-giving oxygen into your cells. But as you process

Folk remedy offers tangy relief

Vinegar is an old-time treatment for the pain and swelling of all forms of arthritis. Even now, some people swear by it. Try mixing 1 teaspoon each of apple cider vinegar and honey into a glass of water and drinking before meals.

that oxygen, you also produce substances called free radicals, unstable molecules that travel throughout your body damaging healthy cells. This is called oxidation. The more free radicals, the more oxidation – a nasty state of affairs because the cells of your body become weak and prone to disease. Luckily, your body also produces antioxidants, which turn free radicals into harmless molecules. Problems arise, though, when you have too many free radicals and too few antioxidants, due to age or other factors. The good news is you can boost your body's supply of antioxidants through your diet. They naturally occur in many plants, and while you can get several of them in pill form, it's usually best to go to the source.

Eat your way around the color wheel. Some of these antioxidants will be familiar; others may sound a bit strange – vitamin C, beta cryptoxanthin, beta carotene, zinc, zeaxanthin, and vitamin E. But they all help you fight off the damaging effects of rheumatoid arthritis. Most show up in brightly colored fruits and vegetables, so you're going to want to load up your grocery cart with produce like sweet potatoes, broccoli, oranges, papaya, peaches, and bell peppers. What could be better – delicious foods plus a healthier body.

Balance the fats to battle RA pain

You may have heard that eating fish, or the omega-3 fatty acids it contains, can keep your heart healthy. But now the hottest news is how people with rheumatoid arthritis can reduce their painful symptoms by getting more omega-3 fatty acids.

These polyunsaturated fats are known to fight inflammation, the process that damages joints and causes pain and swelling in RA. In contrast, omega-6 fatty acids, common in grain-fed red meats and most vegetable cooking oils used in processed and fast foods, bring on more inflammation. If you eat a typical Western diet, you get about 16 times more omega-6 fatty acids than omega-3 fatty acids – not the right balance for healthy joints.

A better mix for people with RA is two or three times as many omega-6 as omega-3 fatty acids. To make this change, limit red meat to around 4 ounces a day and eliminate corn or sunflower oil. Add in lots of cold-water fish, such as salmon and herring, and begin using canola or olive oil. Taking fish oil supplements might also be an option for you – talk to your doctor about side effects and possible drug interactions first. And don't expect immediate relief. The benefits of omega-3 fatty acids might not show up for two to four months.

Bee venom: take the sting out of RA

If you can handle a little sting, you may get some arthritis relief from bee venom. Apitherapy, or the use of honeybee products for healing, has been around since ancient times. Now scientists are testing to see if bee venom is a legitimate arthritis treatment. Studies on rats show a compound in the venom called melittin blocks a natural enzyme, cyclooxygenase-2 (COX-2), that causes inflammation in your body. You're probably familiar with COX-2 inhibitor drugs, such as celecoxib (Celebrex), that do the same thing.

During treatment, an apitherapist holds a bee to your skin until it stings – up to 100 bees during a single session. Or he mixes bee venom powder with water and injects it. Some people even order live bees from beekeepers so they can treat themselves. You should be careful, however, since many people are dangerously allergic to bee stings.

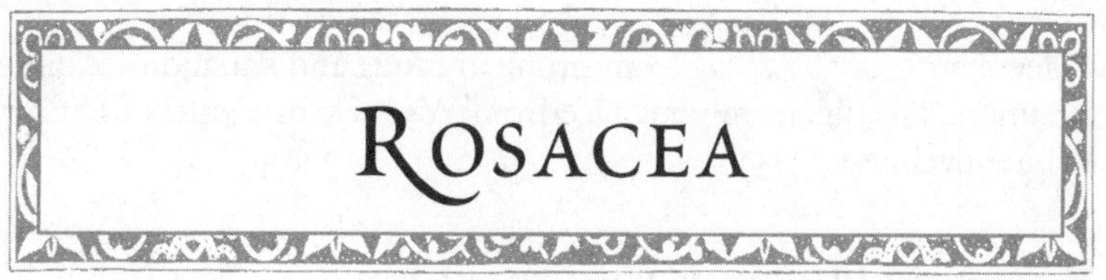

Rosacea

Sure-fire ways to reduce that rosy glow

"His eyes how they twinkled! His dimples how merry! His cheeks were like roses, his nose like a cherry!" With that red face and swollen nose, perhaps good old Saint Nicholas was suffering from rosacea.

Rosy cheeks may make you look healthy, but too much redness in the face can be a sign of this common skin problem. Rosacea usually appears between the ages of 30 and 60 and can last a lifetime. You may tend to blush easily, and you can develop red skin patches, pimples, and thickened skin. Spider veins can appear on your nose and cheeks. The condition also may affect your eyes, making them red, irritated, dry, or watery. It's more common among women, and it tends to hit fair-skinned people of northern or eastern European descent. That's where rosacea gets its nickname, "curse of the Celts."

Many people with rosacea also suffer from migraine headaches. Doctors think both conditions are related to blood vessels that don't expand and contract as they should. Tiny blood vessels in your skin, called capillaries, expand when you blush. With rosacea, these vessels stay stretched, keeping your face red. Rosacea sufferers can expect a flare-up if they eat certain foods, drink hot beverages or alcohol, or spend time in hot or cold conditions. Stress and sun also can bring on trouble. Some doctors suggest taking an 81-milligram baby aspirin once a day to help prevent flushing.

There is no cure for rosacea, but doctors prescribe antibiotic and anti-inflammatory pills and creams to treat the acne, skin infections, and redness. Laser treatments can erase spider veins and correct thickened skin. You can avoid flare-ups by finding your personal triggers and staying away from problem foods and situations. A little attention can transform your face from W.C. Fields redness to Snow White loveliness.

Personal plan keeps rosacea at bay

When it comes to rosacea, everyone is different. Certain foods, drinks, and activities cause flare-ups for some people, but they may not affect others. Common troublemakers include hot or spicy foods, liver, dairy products, some vegetables and fruits, red wine, beer, liquor, and hot drinks like tea and coffee.

A survey found emotional stress is a problem for 91 percent of people with rosacea. Using household sprays with chemicals, like window cleaner, bleach, or even hairspray, also can cause a flare-up. But there is no one-size-fits-all plan, since your personal triggers may differ from those that cause flare-ups in others.

The National Rosacea Society suggests you pay attention to these areas of your life each day to find a link between what you do and when your rosacea acts up.

- What was the weather like? Sunny? Windy? Cold? Hot?
- Did you eat spicy foods?
- What did you drink? Hot coffee or tea? Alcoholic drinks like beer or wine?
- Did you exercise or do physical work like gardening or lifting?
- Were you upset or under stress by something that happened?
- Did you take a hot bath or shower?
- Were you in a heated building?
- What lotions, soaps, makeup, or other products did you use on your face?
- Did you follow your doctor's orders?

Mix up some savory spices

Hot spices like black pepper and cayenne can bring on a rosacea flare-up, but that doesn't have to mean the end of flavorful food. The National Rosacea Society suggests mixing these spices to substitute for troublesome condiments.

Poultry seasoning	½ tsp sage, ½ tsp coriander, ¼ tsp thyme, ⅛ tsp allspice, ⅛ tsp marjoram
Curry powder	4 tsp coriander, 2 tsp turmeric, 1 tsp cinnamon, 1 tsp cumin, ½ tsp basil or oregano, ½ tsp cardamom
Chili powder	2 tsp cumin, 1 tsp oregano

You can get a free diary booklet from the National Rosacea Society to keep track of your personal triggers. Contact the society toll free at 888-NO-BLUSH (888-662-5874) or print a copy from its Web site, *www.rosacea.org*.

Beat the heat to save your skin

Extreme weather – whether cold and windy or hot and humid – can lead to a rosacea flare-up. Hot drinks, hot baths, and too much sun exposure also can bring on a flushing episode, while overheating during exercise is a sure-fire trigger for many people.

Exercise can help reduce stress, yet another common cause of rosacea flare-ups. But don't overdo it. You can get a good workout without causing a flare-up if you follow these tips to keep your cool.

- Exercise during early morning or late evening to avoid the midday sun.
- Find a cool indoor gym instead of exercising in the outdoor heat.

- Wear a hat and use plenty of sunscreen if you must be in the sun.
- Divide a long workout into shorter bursts to avoid overheating.
- Keep a cool, damp towel around your neck.
- Suck on ice chips or drink cold water to lower your body temperature.

Plants provide natural redness relief

Rosacea is a long-lasting problem that can come and go, and some people get tired of using prescription drugs that irritate their skin. Many alternative treatments are available, some promising to soothe redness and inflammation with natural ingredients. Let your doctor know if you use alternative remedies so he can monitor them with your other treatments. Here are three to try.

Prevent symptoms with green tea. Several compounds in green tea have well-known antioxidant and anti-inflammatory actions. Because of this, green tea extract may protect your overly sensitive skin from damaging ultraviolet rays, making you less likely to develop unsightly symptoms. Green tea may also make spider veins less noticeable. Look for skin care products that contain green tea extract in your pharmacy or at the cosmetics counter of your local department store.

MythBuster: Does redness come from alcoholism?

A red-faced, swollen-nosed drunkard is a common figure in literature, comics, and film. In fact, some people still think rosacea is a sign of alcoholism. But people with rosacea are no more likely to drink too much than other folks. Pay attention to your drinking habits if you are prone to rosacea, however, since drinking some kinds of wine, beer, and liquor can bring on a flare-up. A survey of people with rosacea found 52 percent had flare-ups after drinking alcohol.

Battle redness with licorice extract. Researchers tested licochalcone, an extract from the licorice plant's roots, in products for people with reddened skin or rosacea. After eight weeks, their redness improved and their skin problems bothered them less. Try Eucerin Redness Relief skin care system, available at local pharmacies.

Calm irritation with oatmeal. Just as eating oatmeal can calm your nerves, spreading products containing powdered oatmeal on your skin is also soothing. A common ingredient in lotions and other skin care products, oatmeal can fight irritation, itching, and dryness. It even has the endorsement of the U.S. Food and Drug Administration, which calls it a "skin protectant."

Head off problems from eye rosacea

It may surprise you to learn you can have rosacea in your eyes with no signs on the rest of your face. More than half of those with skin rosacea suffer from this serious problem as well.

Watch for symptoms of ocular (eye) rosacea such as redness of your eyelids and whites of your eyes, sensitivity to light, sties on your eyelids, and the feeling that you have dirt or dust in your eye. Your eyes may tear up for no reason, or they may feel dry. Your vision may be blurred, but your contact lenses may be too uncomfortable to wear. Worse, if eye rosacea is not treated, your eyesight can be damaged. It can lead to scarring of your cornea, the transparent tissue covering the front of the eye.

Doctors treat eye rosacea by prescribing antibiotic pills and eye gels, corticosteroid drops, and eye drops to help you make more tears. You can help by keeping your eyes clear of mucous buildup. Try using a watered-down solution of baby shampoo to wash your eyelids every day.

If you have a sty – an infection of a gland on the eyelid – don't try to drain it. That will only spread the infection. Instead, hold a warm, wet washcloth to the sty for a few minutes several times a day until it heals.

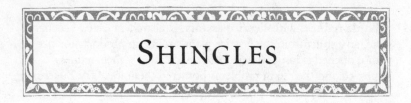

Shingles

Modern remedies overcome ancient affliction

"St. Anthony's fire" is the Italian nickname for shingles, probably because of the burning pain of this common illness. The herpes varicella-zoster virus, which causes chickenpox in children, brings on shingles in adults. After you recover from a bout of chickenpox, the virus lies dormant in your nerve cells. It can reappear years later, usually in older people or those with weakened immune systems.

Shingles is a pain. That's one thing most people with the condition agree on. It often starts with itching, tingling, numbness, or pain along the affected nerve. Sometimes the pain is so sharp people think they have appendicitis or gallstones, and some people think they're having a heart attack.

But a red rash in a band that follows a single nerve along one side of your body – usually the trunk or face – is a sure sign of shingles. In fact, the word shingles is Latin for "belt" or "girdle." Small bumps of the rash develop into fluid-filled blisters before breaking open and crusting over. A case of shingles usually runs its course in about five weeks.

Health professionals say some chickenpox remedies can get you through the pain, itching, and discomfort of shingles. Take aspirin or other nonsteroidal anti-inflammatory drugs (NSAIDs) for pain. Try oatmeal baths, calamine lotion, or antihistamines like Benadryl for itching. To make the blisters feel better, take cool baths or apply cold compresses soaked in Burrow's solution – a drying agent available at drugstores without a prescription.

Most people who come down with shingles get through it with no major problems. But look out for these possible complications.

Eye problems. A shingles rash on the tip of your nose, called Hutchinson's sign, means the virus probably is affecting the nerves of your eye. If your eye is involved, you may have a serious infection that can damage your eyesight.

Ramsay Hunt syndrome. Shingles in your ears or mouth can cause facial paralysis, ear pain, hearing loss, ringing in your ears, nausea, vomiting, loss of taste, and dizziness. The hearing loss usually clears up, but facial paralysis may not.

Postherpetic neuralgia (PHN). Shingles rash is just the beginning of problems for some people. Lingering pain caused by nerve damage can last for months after the rash clears up.

See your doctor at the earliest sign of a shingles outbreak. Antiviral drugs can keep the disease from becoming more serious, but they work best if you start taking them within three days of getting shingles. Other drugs can help you avoid or deal with complications.

You can't give shingles to another person, since it must be reactivated from a virus that's been hiding in your nerve cells. But you can spread the virus in the form of chickenpox to someone who hasn't had that disease. If you live to be 85 years old, you have a 50-percent chance of having shingles. But there's good news. A new shingles vaccine is available for seniors. And that's not all – lifestyle changes, like eating more fruits and veggies and getting regular exercise, may help you head off shingles.

Vitamin and mineral combo defeats virus

Researchers in England found eating a diet rich in fruits and vegetables – or taking a special blend of vitamins and minerals – helped people avoid shingles by boosting their immune systems.

Vitamin A, vitamin B6, vitamin C, vitamin E, folic acid, iron, and zinc were studied in two groups of people – those with shingles and those without. Researchers believe these vitamins and minerals work together to create stronger immunity against shingles. No improvement was seen when people took just one of the seven nutrients.

People in the study who didn't get enough of the nutrients were five times more likely to get shingles.

The study also showed that people who ate less than one serving of fruit a week had three times the chance of developing shingles than people who ate more than three servings a day.

Traditional Chinese exercise heads off shingles

Not everyone who had chickenpox gets shingles as an adult. As you age, your body has fewer immune cells to ward off the herpes varicella-zoster virus, so you're more likely to come down with the painful condition. However, research shows a traditional form of exercise can keep your immunity level high and ward off shingles.

Tai Chi Chih, a form of Chinese exercise sometimes called "meditation with movement," is a type of martial art developed for seniors. It uses a series of 20 poses and slow movements in a particular sequence.

Experts in California gathered a group of 18 seniors and had them take 45-minute Tai Chi Chih classes three times a week for 15 weeks. They tested the levels of immune cells specific to shingles in the seniors before and after the study. Then the researchers compared these people with a group of seniors who did not take the Tai Chi Chih classes.

The exercising seniors could boast of a 50-percent increase in their immunity against shingles. That means the exercise poses may help prevent a painful shingles attack. It's possible Tai Chi Chih's ability to lower stress is the reason it strengthens immunity. People in the classes also did better in their everyday movements, like walking and climbing stairs. Those in the control group, who did not take the classes, did not improve their immunity or movement.

DIY remedies cream PHN pain

Mothers treat chickenpox in their children with soothing oatmeal baths and calamine lotion. The same tricks may work for the itching and discomfort of a shingles rash.

But the long-lasting pain of postherpetic neuralgia (PHN) calls for a different treatment. About 10 to 20 percent of people who get shingles get PHN, defined as pain that lingers for more than a month after the rash clears up. Experts think it comes from damage to your nerves by the virus. Your doctor can prescribe drugs, but you may find relief from topical treatments.

Capsaicin, the natural chemical that makes chili peppers taste hot, blocks pain when you rub it on your skin. It binds to nerve receptors in your skin, causing a bit of irritation at first. After a while, capsaicin makes the receptors less sensitive so your skin doesn't transmit the pain and irritation signals. Although you can make your own capsaicin cream from chili peppers and olive oil, it's easier and safer to buy a tube of capsaicin cream, like Zostrix or Capzasin-HP. Just

MythBuster: What if you're surrounded?

A popular folk belief says if a shingles rash wraps around your body and meets, you'll die. Since shingles nearly always affects the nerves on only one side of your body, this meeting is rare. That's why people must have been scared when it happened. In fact, fewer than 1 percent of people with shingles have the rash on both sides. Although having shingles on both sides is more serious, you probably won't die from being surrounded. You can skip the old-time advice to tie an eel skin around your waist to keep the rash from meeting.

Arm yourself against shingles

Zostavax , a new vaccine to prevent shingles, was approved in 2006. It's a more powerful form of the chickenpox vaccine, which children have been getting since 1995. Zostavax can cut in half your risk of getting shingles. Even if you develop shingles after you get the vaccine, you'll have less discomfort and a lower chance of suffering the serious, lingering pain of postherpetic neuralgia (PHN).

The vaccine may seem a bit pricy at $150, but a study found having shingles can be much more expensive. Using health insurance records of people across the United States, researchers found a typical case of shingles costs about $430 – even more for seniors and those with complications. Most of that money goes for doctor visits and drugs. Health insurance should help pay for the vaccine, which is included under Medicare's Part D prescription program.

The shingles vaccine is for people 60 years and older. People with weakened immune systems from cancer treatments, organ transplants, or other causes may not be good candidates for the vaccine.

remember – capsaicin cream may not help for the first six weeks, and don't use it until your blisters are completely dry.

Topical salicylates (Aspercreme) or creams with menthol (Flexall 454), from the peppermint plant, may also help deaden PHN pain. If these don't work, your doctor may prescribe a patch containing topical lidocaine or prilocaine.

PHN can be frustrating, but take hope from knowing it usually goes away within three months.

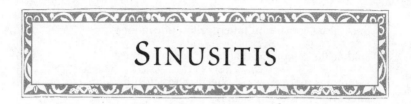

Sinusitis

Breathe easier at last

Recognizing when you have sinusitis can be like an episode of "To Tell the Truth." The symptoms of sinusitis are so similar to the signs of colds, flu, and allergies that you may find yourself saying, "Will the real troublemaker please stand up?" The secret is to get savvy about sinuses so you can help yourself.

Your sinuses are open pockets in your skull that lie behind your forehead and on either side of your nose. They connect to your nasal passages. In fact, they produce mucus to grab and remove harmful bacteria and pollutants from your nose and sinuses.

Normally, mucus is thin, and the tiny hair-like cilia along your sinus and nasal passages can move it along. But colds, flu, low indoor humidity, or hay fever can inflame the lining of your nasal passages and sinuses. That inflammation is called sinusitis. It makes your sinuses and nasal passages drier and swollen. The added dryness may thicken the mucus so you get a stuffy nose and your cilia can't sweep out harmful bacteria and irritants. And, if the swelling blocks the opening that allows your sinuses to drain, you get sinus pain and pressure, too.

Even worse, bacteria from your nasal passages sometimes sneak into your sinuses. Clogged sinuses are the perfect place for bacteria to multiply like rabbits, so occasionally sinusitis becomes a bacterial sinus infection.

Stuffy nose, sore throat, coughing, and facial pressure are common signs of colds, allergies, and sinusitis. But if the following symptoms develop, see a doctor because you may have a sinus infection.

- thick nasal congestion tinted yellow, green, or gray
- cold or flu symptoms that last 10 days or longer
- symptoms that get worse after five to seven days or return soon after you start feeling better
- high fever and sudden or severe illness
- face or tooth pain, especially when you bend over

Your doctor will determine whether you need an antibiotic for a bacterial infection. But if a virus caused your sinusitis, antibiotics won't help. Fortunately, your doctor can recommend other medications to ease your symptoms. She can also find out whether you have acute sinusitis or the chronic version. Acute sinusitis vanishes within 30 days, but chronic sinusitis either fades and comes back repeatedly or lasts at least three months.

If you have chronic sinusitis, your doctor may refer you to a specialist. He can nab or rule out underlying conditions like allergies, asthma, immune problems, gastraoesophageal reflux disorder (GERD), and structural blockages. He can also check your mucus for fungi. Some people with chronic sinusitis have intense allergic and inflammatory reactions to fungi and may need different medication.

Once you know what is wrong, you can start fighting back. If you have allergies, for example, see the *Hay fever* chapter. But if you have sinusitis try these.

- Give your cilia a hand. Flush your nasal passages regularly with the irritant-removing rinse found in the *Hay fever* chapter.
- Using a drug-free saline nasal spray twice a day can mean fewer days with a runny or stuffy nose, research shows. Save the empty bottle if you buy your first spray from a drugstore. Mix a refill from 8 ounces of warm water and a half teaspoon of salt.
- Sleep with your head slightly raised to help your sinuses drain. If one side is stuffier than the other, sleep with that side tilted

Avoid a vicious cycle

Decongestant nose sprays like Afrin may work wonderfully for the first few days. But your body builds up a tolerance against them after that, and they may cause your nasal passages to swell. Using the spray more often only helps for a little while. The more often you take the spray, the more your body resists its effects until the nose spray simply stops working. But you can avoid this vicious cycle if you stop using these sprays after three days and switch to a saline spray instead.

down. Avoid sleeping too much or too little, too. Both can aggravate your sinuses.

- Try exercise. Even a simple walk can help clear nasal passages for most people.
- Drink at least six glasses of liquids daily. That helps keep your mucous membranes moist, so they can keep defending you against harmful bacteria. Water is your best bet, but you can also enjoy herbal teas, diluted fruit juices, and thin soups.

Moisture makers unblock sinuses

Painless sinuses could be just a stove pot away. That's because steam and mist are surprisingly good at unclogging stubborn sinuses. They thin the thick mucus to help ease sinus pressure, pain, and stuffiness. All you have to do is pick your favorite way to get all steamed up.

Take a hot shower. Keep the steam from escaping by closing the bathroom door and windows before you start. If you don't have time for a shower, use a facial sauna or steam inhaler instead.

Make a miniature steam tent. Bring water to a boil and turn the heat down. Don't breathe the steam while the water is boiling. It could damage the tender membranes in your nose and make things worse. Instead, after the boiling stops, put a towel over your head, lean over the steaming pot, and breathe in the warm vapors for 15 minutes. For more unclogging power, add a few drops of eucalyptus oil or peppermint oil to the water. These oils have anti-inflammatory properties and may boost the sinus-draining effect of the steam.

Steam or mist nightly. Run an inexpensive cool-mist humidifier or warm-mist vaporizer in your bedroom during the night. Keep all bedroom doors and windows closed. For best effects, start the humidifier or vaporizer a few hours before bed, and close up the room to let the humidity levels build to sinus-soothing levels. Clean the unit regularly with vinegar and water to prevent the molds that cause sinus infections.

Pungent spices bring speedy relief

Spice up your favorite soup and start eating. Soon your painful, clogged sinuses will empty and you'll feel much better. That's because seasonings like cayenne, horseradish, ginger, and garlic help thin your mucus and end the pain. Hot sauce or Cajun spice mix work as well.

Add hot spices to other dishes or just stick with chicken soup. This soup has anti-inflammatory powers that may help battle the sinus infection even after the spices wear off. Just remember these warnings:

- Add only as much spice as you're comfortable eating.
- Don't try fiery spices if they give you heartburn.
- Avoid these spices if you have an ulcer, chronic heartburn, or gastroesophageal reflux disease.

Hot compresses cool the misery

A hot compress could be just the thing to ease your misery, and it's easy to prepare. Just dampen a small pile of washcloths or towels with hot water. Use hot tap water, or heat wet cloths in the microwave, but don't let the cloths get hot enough to burn you. Wring them out, and

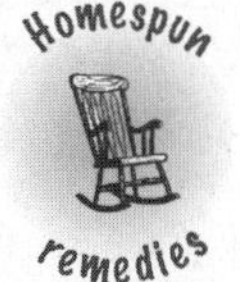

Give your sinuses sweet relief

When your next sinus headache strikes, pop a strongly-scented mint candy like Mentos or Altoids into your mouth. Some people say these sweet treats clear sinus pain and pressure away like magic.

rest them over sinuses that hurt. Place one along your eyebrows, and position the others in the painful places between your eyes and below them. You'll need fresh compresses when these cool, so keep other washcloths warm in an insulated lunch bag, wide-mouthed soup thermos, insulated cooler bag, or crock pot.

Ancient Chinese secret drains away pain

An ancient Chinese art called acupressure might drain your sinuses, and you can do it right in your own home. Just use your fingers to press directly on the inner edges of your eyebrows for a few seconds. Some people actually feel their sinuses start to drain when they do this. Also, try the sides of your nose and the bones below and around your eyes.

Fight sinus clogs with the right foods

Some foods might help slam the door on sinus infections. Find out what to eat and what to avoid.

Fill up on antioxidant-rich foods. People with sinusitis have lower levels of antioxidants in their nasal lining than everyone else, a Danish study suggests. Those antioxidants may help neutralize free radicals, the harmful molecules that may contribute to your sinus problems. Antioxidants may also help rev up your immune system to fight off colds and sinus infections. To get more antioxidants, eat foods with plenty of vitamin C, vitamin A, beta carotene, and glutathione. Good choices include asparagus, avocado, broccoli,

MythBuster: Can milk irritate sinuses?

Milk won't make your sinus symptoms worse, research shows. Dairy products can only create congestion if you have an allergy or intolerance to them. But if you already have symptoms, milk isn't your best bet for getting more fluids. Make sure you're drinking plenty of water, diluted juices, and other hydrating beverages before you fill up on milk.

cantaloupe, kale, sweet potatoes, sweet peppers, carrots, papaya, and spinach. Some experts recommend vitamin supplements, but talk to your doctor to determine whether you need them.

Eat a balanced diet. To further fortify your battered immune system, eat far more servings of produce, whole grains, beans, and nuts than meats, dairy, salty foods, and sugary treats. Enjoy fish once or twice a week, too. But gradually cut back on caffeine until your total is two drinks or less daily. Caffeine helps dehydrate your body and may increase the amount of mucus your body makes.

Drink your probiotics. People who drank a probiotic daily for a month reduced the number of sinus-infecting bacteria lurking in their nasal passages, researchers say. Yogurt contains a different probiotic and didn't have the same effect. Studies suggest foods containing *Lactobacillus GG* are your best bet. Try Danimals or a similar product.

Check for hidden food allergies. An undiscovered allergy to a particular food or drink can cause sinus congestion or make your sinusitis worse. If you already suspect a food like milk, avoid it for a week or two to see if your symptoms improve. Other potential allergy-causers include shellfish, nuts, tomatoes, soy, peanuts, wheat, rye, oats, chocolate, corn, oranges, dairy products, eggs, and artificial food coloring. If eliminating all these isn't practical, see an allergist for testing.

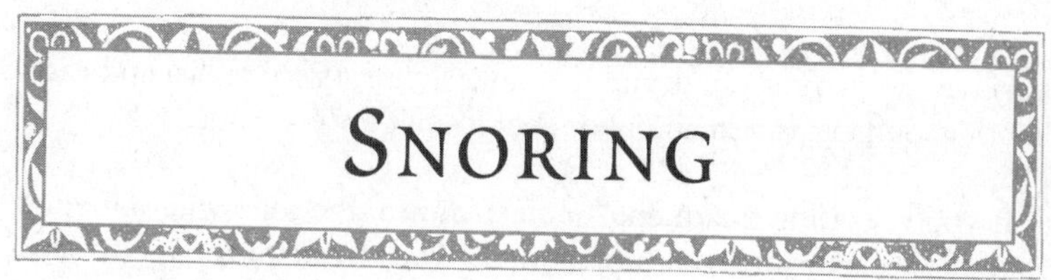

Snoring

Great strategies for a 'silent night'

Snoring doesn't just prevent you from getting a good night's sleep. It can also raise your risk of heart disease, auto accidents, diabetes, and an unhappy spouse. But before you buy one of the hundreds of pricey snoring remedies, find out what causes it and what you can do about it – cheaply and naturally.

During sleep, certain triggers may relax the muscles in your airway so much that your throat narrows. That can restrict or block the flow of air when you breathe and may even create air turbulence in your throat. The turbulence may vibrate your tongue and soft palate – the divider that separates your breathing passage from the passage leading to your stomach. That vibrating makes the snoring sound.

So what makes one person more prone to snoring than another? Some people have a long soft palate that encourages snoring. Others only snore when allergies, colds, or sinus problems make normal breathing difficult. Getting older or heavier raises your odds of snoring. But for an unlucky few, loud snoring may be a sign of a serious condition called sleep apnea.

People with sleep apnea often stop breathing during sleep. After 10 to 60 seconds, they awaken briefly to start breathing again, but rarely remember waking. If you snore heavily no matter what position you sleep in, if your snoring disturbs your family, or if your spouse says you struggle to breathe while asleep, talk to your doctor about sleep apnea.

No store-bought remedy can cure sleep apnea. Fortunately, your doctor can recommend a mouth guard, special pillows, or the continuous positive airway pressure device to painlessly treat sleep apnea and ease snoring. Surgery is also an option, but it's not for everyone.

If you're getting treatment for sleep apnea, the following remedies may reduce snoring even more. And if you're one of the many snorers who does not have sleep apnea, these secrets may silence your snoring for good.

Lose pounds to win the snore war

Not only can weight gain cause snoring but snoring may also cause weight gain. Here's how it works. As you gain weight, fatty deposits build up in your neck and press against your throat. That constricts your airway and encourages snoring. Snoring disrupts your sleep and leads to another problem.

Sleep loss revs up the hormones that trigger your appetite. If you eat more and gain extra weight, your snoring could get worse. If that causes more sleep loss, your appetite could grow, leading to more pounds and more snoring. The sooner you can stop this vicious circle, the better off you'll be. The good news is losing weight reduces the fat deposits that restrict your airway. As the pressure relaxes, your snoring and sleep improve, and your appetite-stimulating hormones return to normal. That might be enough to permanently keep the weight off and the snoring away.

Simple tactics unstuff a stuffy nose

You've probably wondered why a stuffy nose makes you snore and how you can stop it. When colds, allergies or sinusitis stuff up your nose, you work harder to pull air in. The extra effort creates a vacuum in your throat and narrows your airway, which promotes snoring. Here's what you can do about it.

Turn pro. The nasal strips professional football players wear may relieve snoring. Research shows they make breathing easier for people with stuffy noses, and the National Sleep Foundation suggests they're worth a try.

Be a quitter. Smoking makes nasal congestion worse. Quit to breathe easier and snore less.

Get steamed. Close up the bathroom and take a steamy shower before bed. The steam thins out the thick mucus that's stuffing up your nose. If you can't shower, pour hot water in a bowl, put a towel over your head, lean over the bowl, and breathe in the steam for 15 minutes. If you need something stronger, close up your bedroom and run an inexpensive warm-mist vaporizer or cool-mist humidifier during the night. Just remember to clean the unit regularly.

4 ways to say good night to snoring

Try these tips to improve your sleep and cut down on complaints from the other side of the bed.

Sleep like a spaceman. Research with astronauts suggests gravity makes your airway sag backward when you recline. That blocks the flow of air and causes snoring. Although you can't get rid of gravity, using blocks to elevate the head of your bed could prevent your airway from sagging.

Watch your back. Sleeping on your side instead of your back may do wonders, too. To keep from rolling on to your back, tuck a pillow behind you. Or sew a deep pocket on the back of a pajama shirt, put a tennis ball in it, and sleep in the pajamas.

Don't drink and sleep. Avoid alcohol for the last four hours before bedtime. Alcohol relaxes your tongue and throat muscles, which narrows your airway and triggers snoring.

Be wise about Rx. Medications that make you sleepy, like tranquilizers, antihistamines, and sleeping pills, can also relax your airway and make snoring more likely. If you think a drug you're taking is causing you to snore, talk with your doctor. But never stop taking a drug your doctor prescribed without his approval.

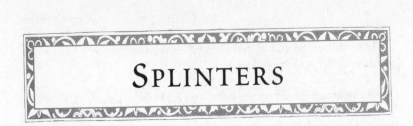

Splinters

Give painful slivers the slip

According to a startling folk remedy, a simple way to get a splinter out of your foot is to keep it near a bag of hot manure all night. Fortunately, there are better ways to get rid of splinters. Here's what you need to know.

Splinters happen when a sliver of something punctures your skin and decides to stick around. These sneaky slivers usually jab into your hand or foot, where they can cause the most aggravation. Even worse, splinters usually bring dirt and germs along for the ride. Your best bet is to get the splinter out before it triggers an infection or allergic reaction. The best way to do that often depends on the splinter.

Some splinters are painless because they barely pierce the skin, while others stab deeply, hurt a lot, and may even bleed. You can remove most splinters yourself, but see a doctor if any of these apply to you.

- The splinter is deep in your skin and would be difficult to remove.
- You cannot get the splinter out.
- The splinter site shows signs of infection, like redness, swelling, tenderness, puffiness, pain, bleeding, or pus. These could be warning signs that part of the splinter is still in your skin.
- You have fever, swollen lymph glands, and red streaks on your skin pointing from the splinter toward your heart.
- You cannot easily remove a splinter under your fingernail or toenail.
- The splinter is very large or has a barbed end.

- Your last tetanus shot was more than five years ago. Ask your doctor about getting this shot every five years.

You might be surprised to learn that wood isn't the only source of splinters. You can also get them from glass, metal, plastic, and thorny or spiny plants. Tweezers can remove most splinters, but you'll discover safer tricks for tiny plant stickers, fiberglass, and tiny painless splinters later in this chapter.

Meanwhile, if your splinter doesn't fit those categories, here's a great way to remove it. Clean around the area with soap and water, but don't soak a wooden splinter because water makes wood swell.

Sterilize a needle and a pair of tweezers with rubbing alcohol. If you can't grasp the top end of the splinter with tweezers, numb the area with an ice cube. Then make gentle cuts in the skin near the top of the splinter with the needle until more of the splinter is exposed.

Position the tweezers close to the skin and slant them so you can pull out the splinter from the same angle it entered. Grasp the splinter with the tweezers and remove it. Then clean the area with soap and water and apply antibacterial ointment.

3 pain-free ways to pluck splinters

Tiny splinters from plants like cactus or stinging nettle may break apart if you use tweezers to grab them. Tweezers may also be a poor choice for fiberglass splinters and shallow, painless splinters. Try these simple remedies instead.

- White glue. The same glue you used for arts and crafts in kindergarten could smoothly slide your splinters out. Just cleanse the splintered area, apply a layer of glue over it, and let the glue dry. Peel off the glue and say goodbye to your splinters. But don't try this trick with super glue. It won't work and could be dangerous.

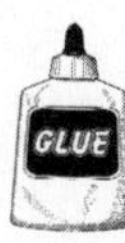

- Facial gel or hair removal wax. Use this the same way as white glue, but be ready to use tweezers to help peel the layer after it dries.

- Tape. Lightly press a layer of clear tape over the splintered area and then pull it off. You'll probably spot splinters on the tape. Clear packing tape is your best bet, but other transparent tapes may also work if they're very sticky.

Epsom salt 'draws out' the invader

That splinter under your skin might come out without a needle. According to the Epsom Salt Industry Council, a compress of Epsom salt may draw the splinter to the surface. Epsom salt pulls sweat and toxins out of your pores and up to the skin's surface, so a splinter might come along for the ride. If you have a new splinter that shows no redness, pus, swelling, or other signs of infection, try this before you break out the needle. Mix one-fourth cup of Epsom salt in two cups of very warm water. Dip an absorbent cloth in the mixture, wring it out, and rest it over the splinter for 15 minutes.

Baking soda works like magic

Try this clever trick to make a splinter slide out on its own. Mix a teaspoon of baking soda with enough water to make a thick paste. Gently spread the paste over your splinter and cover it with an adhesive bandage. Just make sure you don't press hard enough to push the splinter in further. After two hours, remove the bandage and rinse off the paste. Check for your splinter but don't be surprised if it's missing in action.

SPRAINS & STRAINS

Stamp out pain and swelling

In northern England, people born breech could supposedly cure sprains and strains by stamping on them. The hurt person stretched their injured limb out on the ground for the "healer" to stomp on. Afterward, the folk healer wrapped the wound in eel-skin bandages to finish healing. Luckily, this remedy has fallen out of fashion, although a good stomping would surely take your mind off the pain of a strain.

Sprains happen when you stretch or tear ligaments, the soft tissue that ties together the bones in your joints. Strains occur when you stretch or tear muscles or tendons, the tissue connecting your muscles to your bones.

Anything that stretches a joint out of place, like falling on it at an odd angle, twisting it, or getting hit can cause a sprain. Wrists, ankles, and knees are all common spots for injury. Strains, on the other hand, can either strike suddenly or develop over time. You could strain your back while lifting something the wrong way or get a chronic strain from doing the same movements day after day. Your back is a prime spot for strains, as are your hands, arms, elbows, and hamstring, the muscle that runs along the back of your thigh.

Both types of injury cause swelling and pain. The worse your symptoms, the more severe your injury. Take a look on the following page at how to tell whether you have a sprain or strain.

Sprain symptoms	Strain symptoms
bruising	muscle spasms
trouble moving or using a joint	trouble moving a muscle
feeling a pop or tear when the injury happens	muscle weakness

As soon as you hurt yourself, your body goes to work repairing the damage. The injured cells release chemicals that make the area inflamed. Blood vessels widen, rushing nutrient-rich blood to the injury site. White blood cells tear down and cart away damaged tissue, clearing the way for scar tissue to form. As it does, you regain strength in the injured area. Within a month or so, the scar tissue may start shrinking, drawing the torn tissue back together.

You can treat most sprains and strains at home with the advice in this chapter. However, you should see a doctor immediately if:

- you are in extreme pain.
- you can't move the injured joint or put any weight on it.

Antibiotics linked to serious injuries

Like the arrow in his heel that killed him, you can bet the great Achilles never saw this danger coming. Quinolone antibiotics, such as ofloxacin (Floxin), ciprofloxacin (Cipro), and norfloxacin (Noroxin), weaken your Achilles tendon, the tissue connecting your calf muscle to the back of your heel. If you are over the age of 60, these antibiotics can make you more likely to rupture your Achilles tendon, especially if you also take corticosteroids. If you sprain your ankle while taking quinolones, see your doctor. It could be a much more serious injury.

- the injured area looks crooked or has lumps and bumps that aren't from swelling.
- you notice numbness, coolness, or discoloration.
- you injure the same joint or muscle you've hurt before.
- you aren't sure how serious the injury is or how to treat it.

First aid for common injuries

The early swelling of a sprain or strain may feel tender and painful, but it's necessary for healing. However, if the inflammation continues unchecked, it can slow your recovery. That's why it's important to follow the RICE rules as soon as you suffer an injury.

Rest. Give your body a rest. Stay as active as you can, but avoid putting weight or pressure on the injury for two days. Skip activities that cause pain.

Ice. Ice down the area as soon as you hurt it. Cold numbs pain but also constricts blood vessels, limiting blood flow to the area and putting a cap on inflammation. Plus, if you have torn any tissue, the ice will help stop internal bleeding. Apply ice for 20 minutes at a time, four to eight times a day for the first few days, then as needed for swelling. People with diabetes or circulation problems should talk to their doctor before using ice therapy.

Compression. Wrap the injured joint with elastic bandages to help relieve swelling. Just be sure not to bind it too tightly and cut off circulation. Start wrapping farthest from your heart and move inward. Loosen the bandages if the pain gets worse, the area becomes numb, or the injury starts swelling below the bandage.

Elevation. Prop the injured area up higher than your heart, especially at night, to reduce swelling. Gravity helps drain the extra fluid.

Doctors also recommend taking a nonsteroidal anti-inflammatory drug (NSAID) like aspirin, ibuprofen (Advil, Motrin IB), or naproxen

(Aleve) to control inflammation and pain. After two or three days, you can use heat – hot soaks or heating pad – to relax your muscles. But wait until the swelling goes down. Heat can worsen swelling and internal bleeding because it opens up blood vessels, increasing blood flow to the injured area.

Herbal rubs bring on relief

Menthol, comfrey, and arnica – these three herbal ingredients give many pain relief rubs their power. Here's why.

Menthol, the active ingredient in peppermint oil, activates the cold sensors in your skin, which blocks pain signals from traveling to your brain.

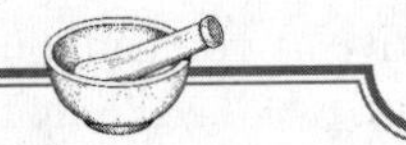

For a super-relaxing soak, dissolve 2 cups of Epsom salts in a tub of hot water. These salts boost circulation and are rich in magnesium, a mineral that helps heal muscles. They're also natural astringents, said to ease swelling and shrink inflamed tissue. Diabetics and other people with dry or fragile skin should avoid soaking in Epsom salts, since they may cause excessive dryness.

Folk healers have traditionally rubbed comfrey ointments on the skin to help heal wounds, and experiments show this herb is a powerful anti-inflammatory. Ointments and creams have reduced swelling, eased pain, and improved movement in people with strains and sprains. Experts say this herb contains cancer-causing agents and can damage the liver, so don't rub it on broken skin or use it for more than two weeks.

Long used to treat bruises and swelling, arnica contains compounds called sesquiterpene lactones that make it a natural anti-inflammatory. They prevent cells from making the chemicals involved in inflammation. Use it only as a rub. Arnica can be toxic if swallowed.

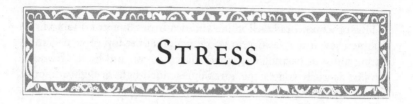

Stress

Learn tension prevention

Stress isn't supposed to make you miserable or sick, but it can. Find out where things went wrong and how you can make them right again.

Think how you'd feel if you saw a car speeding toward you or a grizzly bear in your path. That burst of adrenaline has helped mankind survive predators, natural disasters, and other physical threats. Scientists call it "acute stress" or the "fight or flight response." It temporarily changes your body so you have the extra energy, strength, and peak performance to fight or run from danger. Consider these examples of changes your body makes.

- It starts churning out chemical messengers, including epinephrine (adrenaline) and the stress hormone, cortisol.
- Adrenaline and cortisol raise your heart rate and blood pressure to move blood faster. Your body re-routes blood flow away from less essential organs and sends it to your muscles, brain, and lungs so you'll be ready to run or fight the problem.
- Parts of your immune system are suppressed so their immune fighters can defend the areas of your body where infection or injury is most likely to occur.

Changes like these help you protect yourself until the crisis is over. When you feel safe again, your body's "relaxation response" slashes cortisol and adrenaline levels to reverse the fight-or-flight changes so you can relax and recover.

This process works well in life-and-death situations and rapid-fire emergencies. It may also help you function at the top of your game during a fun or exciting challenge. However, job and home stressors can just as easily trigger the adrenaline-loaded fight-or-flight response. If these stressors persist or if stress is frequent, your stress becomes chronic stress. That means you constantly feel overwhelmed and rarely experience the relaxation response. Instead, continuous exposure to stress hormones prevents you from keeping normal levels of serotonin, the brain chemical that helps you relax. This can make health concerns worse or even lead to many health problems.

☛ High stress can increase memory loss. Research showed that older adults with high stress levels scored up to 50 percent less on cognitive tests – like perception, memory, and judgment – than both older adults with low stress levels and younger adults.

Secrets to stress resistance

Get a good night's sleep and do a fun exercise regularly so you weather stress more easily. Then "vaccinate" yourself against stress with these great ideas.

- Keep friends and family close. People with a strong support network handle stress better.
- Make time for recreation, long weekends, and vacations. These "guilty pleasures" save your family from dealing with your stress-caused illnesses later.
- Writing your worries in a diary may uncover what's causing your stress and reveal new answers to problems.
- Get your doctor's advice on probiotics, helpful bacteria found in fermented milk products like yogurt, and eating well to help manage stress and boost immunity.

- Chronic stress can cripple your immune system, making you more susceptible to colds and other ailments.
- A study of caregivers found that chronic stress also quadruples the levels of inflammation-causing immune factors called cytokines. Increased cytokines have been linked to heart disease, osteoporosis, diabetes, and even some cancers.
- Chronic stress may raise your risk of stroke, ulcers, tension headaches, migraine headaches, sleep problems, and more.

You're more likely to experience chronic stress if you're an older adult, a working mother, or a caregiver for a disabled or ill family member. You may also be at higher risk if you're divorced, widowed, or have money problems. Fortunately, stress management and over-the-counter medicines, like aspirin, antacids, and anti-diarrhea medicines, can often ease stress and its side effects. Nevertheless, if your symptoms get worse or awaken you at night, see your doctor.

Symptoms of stress can also resemble anxiety disorders or depression. If you experience fear, apprehension, or panic even when threats or stressful conditions are absent or if you've had feelings of sadness, hopelessness, loss of interest in your life, or thoughts of suicide, see your doctor for help.

If you're facing chronic stress, consider this. Some stressors can't be avoided, but stress management can help you cope. What's more, the tips in this chapter may help you find solutions to your problems and get stress back under control.

Coping skills help you maintain your cool

You can insulate your mind against stress just as you insulate your house against the cold. Here's how.

Plan for the worst. If you're worried about an upcoming event, ask yourself what are the worst things that could happen. For each possibility, make a plan to prevent it and a second plan for how you'll manage if it happens anyway.

Hope for the best. Research suggests positive coping skills like these help people stress less.

- When faced with a bad situation, find something good about it.
- Instead of calling a difficulty a "problem," label it a "challenge."
- When you're down or worried, count your blessings.

Rate your chances. If you're stressing about something that might occur, ask yourself, "Would a Las Vegas odds maker give this good odds of happening?"

Add your own laugh track. Watch and read more things that make you laugh out loud. Or the next time you're in stressful circumstances, imagine how a comedian would describe it. Research shows that laughter lowers your levels of cortisol and other stress hormones. It also releases tension, helps you keep your perspective, and boosts your immune system.

Take the test of time. Ask yourself, "Will this matter 10 years from now?"

Move on from grudges. Anger and resentment contribute to stress. In fact, holding a grudge means the person who caused the grudge has power over your state of mind. Research shows people who release their grudges feel better emotionally and physically. Seek out positive things to say about the event that caused the grudge. Then resolve to let go of your resentment, so the grudge-causer won't have power over you anymore.

Try prayer. Prayer can lead to positive emotions that may lower your stress hormones. Besides, you can do it anywhere and anytime.

Focus on the important stuff. When you're distressed, think about the things that are most important to you, such as religion, social issues, or personal values. Research shows doing this lowers your cortisol levels.

2 easy ways to tame tension

You might be surprised to learn you can make the relaxation response happen anytime you want. In fact, here are two ways to call on relaxation anywhere without spending a penny.

Deep breathing exercises. During stress, you naturally take rapid, shallow breaths from your chest. Relaxed breathing comes from your diaphragm, just below your chest. Try this. Rest one hand on your stomach. Then inhale slowly and deeply through your nose while counting from one to four. You should feel your stomach rise or move outward. Exhale as you count backward from four to one and feel your stomach sink or move inward.

Repeat this breathing five or 10 times to feel tension drain away. If possible, do these breathing exercises several times daily.

Progressive muscle relaxation. Progressive muscle relaxation relaxes your body one muscle group at a time. Sit or lie down before you start.

Begin by clenching or tightening the muscles of your toes while you count to 10. Then relax them for a count of 10. Notice how heavy and warm they feel – like sinking into your bed at the end of the day.

Repeat this tensing and relaxing with the muscles of your feet. Then

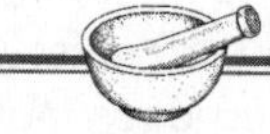

Look no further than lavender for stress relief. Long used for relaxation, this tiny purple flower can help ease anxiety and melt your cares away. Try this quick remedy. Add five to 10 drops of lavender essential oil to a hot bath, along with 1 ounce of carrier oil, like almond, apricot, or jojoba. For a treat for your feet, add a few drops of lavender to a foot bath and soak for 10 minutes.

continue up your body, tensing and relaxing each muscle group. Be sure to include your calves, thighs, stomach, chest, fingers, hands, arms, shoulders, neck, mouth, eyes, and ears. Relaxation will wash over you like a wave, making your tension fade away.

Foods that switch off stress

You could settle for comfort foods, but they are only a temporary fix. What you need are foods that help your mind and body weather stress better over the long haul. Start with these helpful hints.

- Eat a serving of your favorite cereal for breakfast every day. Research suggests this may help you hold down your levels of the stress hormone, cortisol.
- Load up on antioxidant-rich fruits and vegetables and you might prevent stress from raising your risk of illness. Stress makes your body produce more of the harmful free radical molecules that help cause disease. Antioxidants neutralize free radicals and defend your immune system.
- Enjoy produce that's high in vitamin C, such as strawberries, oranges, sweet peppers, kiwi fruit, and broccoli. You need this vitamin to make serotonin and control your cortisol levels.
- Get more of yummy foods like bananas, sweet potatoes, spinach, chicken breast, and baked potatoes. These foods are rich in vitamin B6, a vitamin that helps raise your brain's serotonin levels so you can relax.
- Cookies, white bread, sugar-loaded drinks, snack cakes, white rice, and other sugary or starchy carbohydrates are the kind of fiber-free foods that leave you tired and lifeless. Instead, seek out high-fiber carbohydrates, like hearty whole grains and mellow sweet potatoes. They keep your energy up and boost your levels of soothing serotonin.
- Twice a week, eat sardines, herring, and other fish rich in omega-3 fatty acids. Researchers found that three weeks of omega-3 supplements reduced the amount of adrenaline and cortisol people

pumped out under stress. But omega-3 supplements aren't safe for everyone, so start eating fish now and ask your doctor how to get more omega-3s.

- People with chronic stress have lower magnesium levels. What's more, magnesium deficiency can spawn symptoms like low mood, tiredness, and confusion – which can make your stress worse. Fight back with high-magnesium foods, like black beans, bran cereal, yogurt, black-eyed peas, and spinach.

Calm coffee jitters and get past tense

Coffee doesn't just give you temporary energy. Research found that people churned out one-third more adrenaline and had more stress on days when they downed caffeine compared to caffeine-free days. All it took to make this happen was the equivalent of three 8-ounce cups of Folgers or one and one-half cups of Starbucks medium coffee. Caffeine can even help trigger panic attacks if you're already prone to them.

Your best bet is to cut back on caffeine, but that may be tricky. Caffeine withdrawal starts 12 to 24 hours after your last cup. If you have a morning coffee every weekday, you'll wake up to withdrawal

Think twice about kava

Herbs can cause side effects and interactions just like drugs. Unlike your prescriptions, most herbs don't carry warning labels, so you may not realize the danger. Take kava, for instance. Widely used to calm anxiety and stress, it seemed promising in studies. But the herb has since been linked to hepatitis, liver failure, muscle weakness, and scaly skin, not to mention dangerous interactions with prescription drugs, such as sleep aids, antidepressants, and alprazolam (Xanax) for anxiety. Experts now strongly warn against using kava, particularly if you have liver disease.

symptoms on Saturday. To fight stress and make your caffeine cutback easier, substitute a cup of black tea for that mug of coffee. In spite of its caffeine content, tea shoves your cortisol levels back down when you're stressed. That can help you relax and bounce back from stress more easily.

Music soothes jangled nerves

Surgery and medical tests can be scary and stressful. Interestingly, people who listened to music while awaiting outpatient surgery had less anxiety than those who didn't. What's more, people who listened to music during an invasive medical test had lower cortisol levels and less fear-related stress. The next time you face a stressful situation, try listening to your favorite music, singing with the radio, or playing your favorite instrument. You may be surprised at how much better you feel.

Extract helps you bounce back

Give your brain a boost. Use this little-known extract for fast relief from stress and mental fatigue. Brand's Essence of Chicken (BEC) is a concentrated liquid extract of chicken meat, but without the fat or cholesterol. According to researchers, college students who took BEC for a week felt more active and less fatigued during stressful exams than other students. The BEC students' blood levels of cortisol also slid back to normal more quickly after stress ended. Animal research suggests BEC raises your serotonin levels and may lead to improvements in both mood and sleep. If you'd like to try BEC, check your nearest Chinese grocery store.

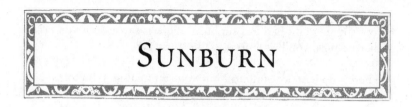

Sunburn

Save your skin while having fun in the sun

Pale skin was once a sign of high social status and wealth. People who worked outdoors showed it on their suntanned or sunburned skin. Ideas changed in the 1920s when French fashion designer Coco Chanel returned from a cruise with dark skin, and the suntan craze began.

Two types of the sun's rays hit your skin. Ultraviolet (UV) B rays are shortwave rays that bring on the redness and blistering of sunburn. UVA rays are long-wave rays that penetrate deeply into your skin to cause long-term problems. Both types cause cells to make free radicals, harmful molecules that lead to skin cancer and photoaging signs, like wrinkles and age spots. People who tan easily because their skin produces lots of melanin when exposed to sunlight have some protection. Fair-skinned people with less melanin are more prone to sunburn.

Some drugs and herbs make your skin more sensitive to the sun so you're more likely to burn, while others can cause a rash or allergic reaction when you're in the sun. Common culprits include diuretics, certain antibiotics like tetracycline, sulfa drugs, high doses of nonsteroidal anti-inflammatory drugs (NSAIDs) used to treat arthritis, some heart and high blood pressure drugs, and the herb St. John's wort.

You can spend time outdoors without risking sunburn. Cover your skin with clothing, use sunscreen, and stay in the shade. A new herbal supplement, Heliocare, may also help. It's made from an extract of a tropical fern, *Polypodium leucotomos.* Early studies show it may work from the inside out, keeping UV rays from damaging cells and causing skin cancer. People who took the supplement before sunning also had less sunburn. Experts say even if you take Heliocare pills, you'll still need to use sunscreen.

There's no cure for sunburn, but you can treat its symptoms with simple home remedies. See a doctor for a more serious sunburn, especially if you have skin blistering, chills, fever, or weakness. Taking precautions to prevent sun damage may help you stay healthy, live longer, and keep your good looks. As Coco Chanel herself said, "A woman has the age she deserves."

Block the burn with timely protection

Prevention is key when it comes to sunburn. It's best to avoid the sun at its midday brightest, from 10 a.m. to 4 p.m. But the sun can do damage at other hours – even on a cloudy day. Try these tips to keep your skin healthy.

Screen out harmful rays. Pick a broad-spectrum sunscreen that shields your skin from both UVA and UVB rays. Your skin type determines which sun protection factor (SPF) you need in your sunscreen. The lighter your skin, the more likely it will burn, and the higher your risk of skin cancer and early wrinkles. You can figure out your skin type by referring to the following chart, developed by Harvard University professor and medical doctor Thomas Fitzpatrick. A lower Fitzpatrick skin type number means you'll need a higher-SPF sunscreen.

Fitzpatrick skin type	Response to sun exposure
I	always burns, never tans, sensitive to sun exposure
II	burns easily, tans minimally
III	burns moderately, tans gradually to light brown
IV	burns minimally, always tans well to moderately brown
V	rarely burns, tans profusely to dark
VI	never burns, deeply pigmented, least sensitive

Some experts suggest using SPF 30 on your face and SPF 15 on the rest of your body. No matter what sunscreen you choose, follow these rules for the best protection.

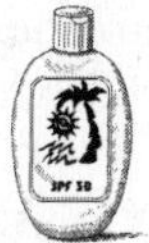

- Use sunscreen every day, even if you plan to be outside for only a short time.
- Slap on lots of sunscreen, and don't skip your ears and feet. About 1 ounce – a shot glass full – of sunscreen is enough to cover your whole body.
- Apply sunscreen 30 minutes before you hit the sun to give it time to be absorbed.
- Reapply at least every two hours and after you swim or exercise.

Stop sunlight cold. Unlike chemical sunscreens, which absorb UV radiation, sunblocks like titanium dioxide and zinc oxide scatter or reflect the sun's rays. They're great for sensitive skin. Old-fashioned sunblocks were thick and white, like the nose creams favored by lifeguards. Some newer types are nearly invisible when you rub them on.

Cover up with clothing. Experts say to wear a wide-brimmed hat and clothing that covers as much skin as possible. Tightly woven fabrics block the most sun, and some have been developed just for sun protection. The FDA approved the Solumbra brand of clothing and hats for SPF 30 sun protection. Find it online at *www.solumbra.com.*

Antioxidants work inside and out

When the sun's rays hit your skin, they start a chemical reaction that creates free radicals. These unstable molecules cause cell damage that can lead to skin cancer, age spots, and other signs of wear and tear on your skin. But you can fight back. Some of the same antioxidant vitamins that prevent other kinds of free radical changes may also fight the skin's signs of aging.

Changing your diet can help. Foods with lots of vitamin A, beta carotene, and other antioxidants may reduce sun damage. Your skin needs vitamin C to produce its main protein, collagen.

One study looked at how your lifetime diet affects your skin. People who ate lots of fruits, vegetables, legumes, eggs, whole grains, nuts, water, and tea showed less sun damage than people who favored whole milk, red meats, butter, potatoes, and sugar.

In another study, researchers tested a high-dose combination of vitamin E and vitamin C supplements to see if they could protect skin from sun damage. After 50 days, people who took the vitamin combo were less likely to sunburn than those who took just one vitamin. Before you try this, check with your doctor. Vitamin and mineral supplements in high doses can have serious side effects.

You can also get antioxidant armor in creams and lotions. Prescription drugs like Retin-A and Renova contain tretinoin, a topical form of vitamin A that works against wrinkles and age spots. But no antioxidants – in food, pills, or creams – can substitute for sunscreen and protective clothing.

First-line treatment: cool, comfort, moisturize

Your sunburn might not show up at first. In fact, it can take four to 24 hours before the redness hits its high note. Then you'll want to treat the pain, protect your skin from infection, and help your sunburn heal.

Rub away the sting. Aloe vera, directly from the plant or in a gel or lotion, is a favorite soother for sunburn. You may prefer creams or lotions with calendula or chamomile, other natural feel-good remedies. Experts don't agree on whether these herbal treatments can make your burn heal faster, but they fight inflammation and ease the pain. Store your lotion in the refrigerator so it cools your skin as you rub it on.

Soak in a cool bath. You can safely add baking soda or colloidal oatmeal to the water to battle pain and itching. Cool compresses also soothe tender skin.

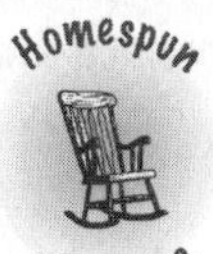

Vinegar puts out the fire

An old-time remedy for sunburn pain is vinegar – white or cider vinegar, diluted in water or applied full strength. Some people say vinegar can take away the sting and turn the red into tan. Add vinegar to a cool bath, drench cloths to make cold compresses, or fill a spray bottle with vinegar to use as needed. Don't use vinegar If your skin is blistered. See your doctor for help.

Take a pain reliever. Over-the-counter drugs like aspirin or ibuprofen help by stopping inflammation and blocking pain.

Drink plenty of water. Severe dehydration can occur if you've been in the sun too long. Symptoms include confusion, anxiety, and sleepiness.

DIY remedies for age spots

Years of fun in the sun can lead to age spots, technically called solar lentigos. These pesky dark spots appear on your hands, face, and other areas exposed to the sun. They look like large freckles and can darken over time. People once thought they were caused by liver disease, so they're sometimes called "liver spots." In reality, they occur when skin cells, damaged by the sun's UV radiation, produce too much pigment. Although age spots are usually harmless, see your doctor to be sure they're not early skin cancer.

Medical treatments to remove age spots include prescription creams or gels like tretinoin (Retin-A) or tazarotene, laser therapy, liquid nitrogen, and chemical peels. These remedies usually do a great job, but they can be expensive. What's more, the drugs can cause side effects. If you're looking for an easier, less-expensive way to lighten your age spots, try these home remedies. Watch for a reaction if you have sensitive skin.

- Use a swab to dab lemon juice on the spots. Natural alpha hydroxy acids in citrus fruits, like lemons, help remove the outer layers of skin cells so new – possibly lighter – cells replace them. Let the lemon juice dry before you go outside, since it makes your skin more sun sensitive.

- Rub on buttermilk – Cleopatra's secret to lovely skin. Like citrus fruits, milk products contain alpha hydroxy acids.
- Mix two parts apple cider vinegar with one part onion juice and paint on the spots in the evening. Leave it to work overnight.

Darker or more stubborn age spots might need stronger treatment, like a fading cream. Over-the-counter products that contain hydroquinone, including Porcelana, Esoterica, and Alpha Hydrox Fade Cream, work slowly over time. They are best for people with light skin because hydroquinone can cause too much bleaching on dark skin. The Food and Drug Administration is considering restricting products with hydroquinone because of fears it may cause cancer. No matter how you get rid of your age spots, protect your skin from the sun so they don't return.

MythBuster: Is sun exposure always bad?

It's wise to avoid baking your skin by sunbathing, but spending some time in the sun is good for you. In fact, you need the sun's UVB rays so your skin can produce vitamin D. Without enough vitamin D, you may be at higher risk for osteoporosis, multiple sclerosis, and certain forms of cancer, like prostate, colon, and breast cancers. You can get vitamin D from foods like tuna, eggs, and fortified milk, but most people get what they need from the sun. Experts suggest getting between 45 minutes and three hours of sun per week depending on your skin color. Keep in mind sunscreen and clothing reduce the amount of sunlight that reaches your skin.

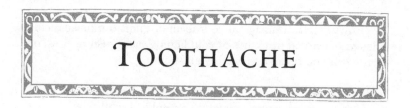

Toothache

Sharp solutions take bite out of tooth pain

"There was never yet philosopher that could endure the toothache patiently" declares an unhappy character in William Shakespeare's *Much Ado About Nothing*. If you've suffered through a toothache, you know the pain can chase all other thoughts from your mind. You want relief, and you want it fast.

Toothaches are the most common mouth pain in adults, and they can make it hard to eat, talk, or swallow. The main causes of toothache include these problems.

Cavities. *Streptococcus mutans* bacteria in your mouth thrive on the starches and sugars in food. As they grow and multiply, these bacteria produce acid that eats through the hard enamel on your teeth to cause decay, or cavities. If the acid eats through to the softer dentin layer, you may feel pain when you eat hot or cold foods. If it reaches your tooth's pulpy center, you'll definitely feel pain.

Tooth abscess. An infection that drains pus into the gums around a tooth forms an abscess. Pain and swelling are sure signs you need a dentist to treat the infection.

Impacted tooth. A tooth that stays below the gum line rather than erupting when it's time can become impacted. This is most common with wisdom teeth since many people don't have enough mouth space for these "third molars."

Sensitive teeth. Damage to your teeth or gums can make them irritated when you drink hot or cold liquids, eat, brush or floss, or even when you breathe through your mouth.

Sinus problems. Sinus congestion may cause pain around your upper teeth – even severe enough to resemble a toothache.

The best way to keep your teeth healthy and free of pain is to eat right and take care of your mouth. The American Dental Association suggests you brush twice and floss once each day, and visit your dentist twice a year.

See your dentist if your tooth pain is severe and doesn't go away in a day or two, or if you have fever or difficulty breathing or swallowing. Your grandma may have applied a vinegar-soaked cloth or smoked a pipe to try to cure her toothache, but you can do better. Untreated tooth decay and infection can spread to nearby bone, skin, and other tissues, even causing death. These serious problems call for serious solutions. If your troubles include dry mouth or gum disease, see those chapters for help.

Head off tooth decay with smart snacking

To prevent cavities, you could rely on help from St. Apollonia, the patron saint of dentistry. A more certain method of keeping your pearly whites both pearly and white is avoiding cavity-causing foods and choosing tooth-healthy snacks. Some foods even keep tooth decay at bay.

Get a craving for cranberry juice. In lab tests, 100-percent cranberry juice prevented cavity-causing *Streptococcus mutans* bacteria from sticking to tooth surfaces. Experts aren't sure why this works, but they think certain flavonols – natural chemicals in the cranberries – do the trick. If the bacteria can't attach to teeth, they can't form plaque in your mouth.

Sip refreshing green tea. An old Chinese saying goes, "When you eat a sweet, drink green tea." Experts have proven this belief is

Worst-choice noshes for healthy teeth

You grew up hearing that candy would rot your teeth, but it's not the only bad boy when it comes to tooth decay. Acidic foods and drinks can also erode your teeth over time, and sugars and starches give bacteria fuel to grow. To protect your teeth, experts say it's best to limit eating and drinking to mealtimes instead of grazing throughout the day.

Drinks to avoid	Foods to avoid
sugary sports drinks	yogurt and other fermented foods
sugar-sweetened sodas	cakes and other sweets
diet sodas	potato chips and french fries
fruit juices	pickles
canned iced tea	citrus fruits

true. Green tea polyphenols help reduce cavities in people who drink the beverage or use green tea extract. Just be sure your tea is not sweetened with sugar.

Dab on some horseradish. Researchers in Japan say isothiocyanates, natural chemicals found in the spicy sushi condiment wasabi, may help protect your teeth from cavities. The chemicals keep cavity-causing bacteria from growing and attaching to teeth. Because real wasabi is expensive, most wasabi served outside of Japan is actually made from horseradish, mustard, and green dye. But researchers say that's fine, since horseradish contains the same isothiocyanates.

See the *Bad breath* chapter for ways these same food items may help banish that problem.

First aid for dental emergencies

Accidents happen. It's a simple fact of life. Sometimes, they involve your teeth. Call your dentist's office immediately for an emergency appointment, and follow this advice.

Handle a knocked-out tooth carefully. Grasp the tooth by the crown, not the roots. Otherwise, you'll damage the living cells needed to reattach it. Gently rinse off any dirt (no scrubbing), and place it inside your cheek to keep it moist until you reach your dentist's office. If you can't hold it in your cheek, wrap it in sterile gauze and submerge it in milk.

Put pressure on a loose tooth. When a tooth gets knocked loose, but not out, try to move it back in place using very light pressure. Don't force it. Bite down to keep it from moving until you arrive at your dentist's office.

Nurse a cracked or broken tooth. Rinse your mouth out with warm water, then apply an ice pack or cold compress to control the swelling. Take ibuprofen, not aspirin, as needed to relieve pain and swelling.

Stay prepared for dental emergencies by keeping a simple first-aid kit on hand. You will need:

- saline solution
- sterile gauze
- handkerchief
- small, lidded container
- ibuprofen
- your dentist's phone number

4 steps to toughen touchy teeth

Smile! If you have sensitive teeth, even grinning for photos can hurt. Exposing your teeth to air, hot or cold drinks, and sticky or acidic foods may trigger an awful ache. Instead of swearing off your favorite foods, start treating the root of your problem.

Get a grip on acid reflux

Gastroesophageal reflux disease, or GERD, causes heartburn and an acid taste in your mouth. That's bad enough, but it can also harm your teeth if it gets out of hand. Strong stomach acid that rises into your esophagus and mouth can erode enamel, the hard surface on the outside of teeth. Over time, chronic GERD can lead to serious, irreversible damage to your teeth. A tooth may look worn, fillings may seem to rise up, and a tooth's pulpy center may be exposed. Ask your doctor about ways to stop acid reflux, like avoiding spicy or fatty foods, taking antacids, or sleeping with your head raised.

Each tooth has several layers. The outer layer, enamel, is the strongest material in your body. It covers and protects the dentin, a layer of tissue full of tiny, hollow tubes. When the enamel wears down or the roots of your teeth become exposed, the dentin loses this protective covering. Then these tiny tubes allow sensations to travel down and jangle the nerves inside your teeth. Luckily, you can take steps to curb this sensitivity and start smiling again.

- Buy soft-bristled brushes, and use a light touch. Scrubbing hard or using hard-bristled brushes can expose your teeth's roots.
- Cut back on diet sodas and acidic foods, including lemon juice, green apples, and kiwi. These can wear away enamel and make your teeth more sensitive.
- Check your current toothpaste. Both whitening and tartar-control toothpastes contain harsh, abrasive ingredients that can aggravate sensitive teeth.
- Ask your dentist about desensitizing toothpastes, like Sensodyne. They contain compounds that block the tubes in dentin, so sensations can't reach the nerves inside. It may take a month or more before you feel a difference.

Urinary Incontinence

Simple tips to beat embarrassing leaks

It's not funny. You suddenly sneezed at a dinner party, and now you're afraid to stand up with a wet spot on your pants. You have urinary incontinence (UI), and you're not alone. The woman across the table has it, too. So does the man at the end.

Fully half of all women develop it. In fact, women are twice as likely as men to have UI, thanks to the rigors of pregnancy and childbirth, menopausal changes, and the way the female body is built. However, men with an enlarged prostate or who undergo prostate surgery may also become incontinent. Brain and nerve damage from strokes, diabetes, or conditions like Alzheimer's disease contribute, too.

Despite how it seems, bladder control problems aren't just a normal part of aging. Experts stress that UI is treatable and often curable, so there's no reason to let it limit your life. Embarrassment is probably your biggest obstacle. In a recent survey, only half of women with UI had even talked about their problem with a doctor. Even fewer – less than a third – were being treated for it.

Your kidneys filter water and waste out of your blood and store them as urine in your bladder. A tube called the urethra carries the urine from your bladder to outside your body. When you urinate, the muscles around your bladder squeeze urine into the urethra. The sphincter muscles surrounding the urethra relax, letting the urine flow out of your body. When you finish, these sphincter muscles contract again, closing off the urethra tightly so urine doesn't escape. When something stops working, you develop one of four types of urinary incontinence.

Stress. If coughing, sneezing, or laughing make you wet your pants, blame it on stress incontinence, the most common kind in women. Your pelvic bone cradles your bladder, and a sheet of muscle called the pelvic floor muscles (PFMs) stretch across the bottom of your pelvic bone to support the bladder. Your urethra drops down through this sheet of muscle.

Being overweight, pregnant, or giving birth can stretch out your PFMs and weaken them. This allows your bladder to drop and push against the bottom of your pelvis. When this happens, the sphincter muscles that keep your urethra closed can't squeeze shut as tightly as they should, so urine leaks out.

Urge. When the need to urinate comes on so fast you can't get to a toilet in time, you probably have urge incontinence. Doctors often call this having an "overactive bladder." Your bladder muscles squeeze at the wrong times, forcing urine out of your body.

Overflow. A bladder that's always full leaks, too. This type of UI tends to strike men more than women. Nerve damage from diseases such as diabetes, or anything that blocks your urethra, like an enlarged prostate, can weaken the bladder muscles so your bladder doesn't fully empty.

Functional. People who are able to control their bladder but have trouble moving or thinking clearly typically have functional incontinence.

The treatment your doctor recommends will depend on what type of UI you have and the severity of your symptoms. She may recommend lifestyle changes, specific exercises, or bladder training. If that doesn't work, she may prescribe medication, special devices, or surgery. You can take a few first steps toward dryness yourself with this advice.

- Eat a high-fiber diet. Fiber fights constipation, a contributor to UI, and helps keep you regular.

- Drink plenty of water. Dehydrating your body actually irritates your bladder, which can worsen UI. Stop drinking fluids two to four hours before bedtime.
- Check your meds. Diuretics, antidepressants, antihistamines, calcium-channel blockers, and beta-adrenergic blockers such as propranolol (Inderal) are just a few drugs that tend to cause urinary incontinence. Talk to your doctor about changing your prescription. Never stop taking a drug your doctor prescribed without his approval.
- Slim down. Being overweight greatly increases your risk of incontinence, especially in women, because it weakens your pelvic floor muscles. Drop those spare pounds with healthy eating and regular exercise.

Special exercise boosts bladder control

Time to tone up those flabby pelvic floor muscles (PFMs). Strengthening your PFMs with special Kegel exercises is one of the easiest ways to improve urinary incontinence in both women and men. In fact, studies show 50 to 75 percent of people who perform Kegels see a major improvement in symptoms, even if they've been incontinent for years.

It's extremely important that you work the right muscles when doing Kegels. Squeezing the wrong ones can actually weaken the muscles that control urination.

- When you urinate, squeeze the muscles that stop the flow of urine. These are the ones you'll use for Kegels.
- Squeeze the muscles you would use to keep from passing gas. You should feel a slight pulling.
- For women, place a finger inside your vagina and tighten your muscles as if you were trying to stop urinating. You should feel a tightening around your finger.

Now that you know how to squeeze, it's time to practice. You can lie down, sit with legs uncrossed, or stand up. Tighten your pelvic floor muscles so you feel a squeeze around both your anus and vagina, for women. Hold this squeeze and count to three, then relax for a count of three. Remember to breathe!

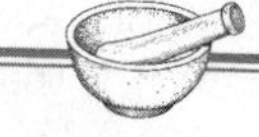

One simple move can stop the most embarrassing episodes of incontinence. Cross your legs or squeeze your urinary muscles when you feel a sneeze or cough coming on. In one study, doing so helped 73 percent of women with stress incontinence hold it in.

Build up to doing this 10 to 15 times, at least three times a day. Do one set of exercises standing, the other sitting, and the last lying down. Alternating positions will make these muscles even stronger. Be careful not to tighten your stomach, thighs, or buttocks while doing Kegels, as this puts more pressure on the muscles controlling your bladder. You may have to exercise faithfully for three to six weeks before your bladder control starts to improve. And keep it up – quit your Kegels, and your incontinence could return.

Bladder training helps end accidents

One of the best ways to thwart stress and urge incontinence is to train your bladder. This helps you control the urge to urinate, wait longer between bathroom trips, and increase the amount of urine your bladder can hold.

Your doctor will probably recommend one of these exercises or a combination of them, depending on your situation. Don't expect instant results. You'll have to work at it for three to 12 weeks. Stay positive when you have accidents and stick with your training.

Learn to hold it. This technique helps you lengthen the time between bathroom trips. When you first feel the urge to urinate, make a conscious effort to hold it for five minutes, then go to the bathroom. When that becomes easy, lengthen your wait to 10 minutes. Ultimately, you only want to go every two to four hours.

Set a schedule. "Bathroom breaks" aren't just for school kids. Create a schedule with the help of your doctor, and try only to go during those set times, even if you don't feel the need to urinate. Start small, perhaps going once every hour, then make your trips further apart until you establish a schedule that works with your bladder's needs.

Gain control. Biofeedback helps you become more aware of your body, so you gain better control over the muscles in your bladder and urethra. A biofeedback trainer will hook you up to a machine that monitors your body and teaches you to control your bladder and urethra to keep them from leaking.

Whatever training method you try, relaxation techniques can help you hold off urinating until your planned bathroom trip. Take deep breaths, do a few Kegel exercises, or distract yourself with television or a good book to take your mind off the urge and make your training a success.

Secret to worry-free workouts

If you're a woman, wearing a tampon may keep you dry during workouts. Tampons push against your vaginal walls, in turn pressing on the urethra. That pressure was enough to prevent leaks while exercising in 86 percent of women with mild stress incontinence. This trick may not work if you have severe incontinence, but it's still worth trying.

Cover the tampon with K-Y Jelly to keep the cotton fibers from sticking to your vaginal walls. You can also shop for specialty tampons made to prevent incontinence. Also, avoid drinking fluids right before you exercise, but be careful not to become dehydrated. Empty your bladder before beginning and take frequent trips to the bathroom during your workout.

UTIs

Turn the tables on urinary tract infections

After the flu and common cold, these infections are the most common reason for visiting a doctor's office. If you're a woman, you can understand why. Three out of five women get a urinary tract infection (UTI) during their lifetimes.

Your kidneys filter water and waste out of your blood, then send it as urine down two thin tubes, called ureters, to your bladder for storage. When you go to the bathroom, your bladder squeezes the urine out through another tube, the urethra. The trouble usually starts when harmful bacteria, such as *E. coli,* from stool contaminate the opening of your urethra. There, they cling and multiply, spreading up the urethra into your bladder, ureters, and even your kidneys if left untreated.

When you urinate, the flow of urine helps wash bacteria out of the urinary tract. Anything that stops or slows the flow, including kidney stones or an enlarged prostate, raises your risk for UTIs. So do conditions like diabetes that weaken your immune system. Wearing a catheter worsens your odds, too, because bacteria on a catheter can easily travel up your urethra. And the simple fact of being a woman puts you at 30 times more risk of UTIs than men.

Most of that higher risk comes from having a shorter urethra – typically one and one-half inches in women, compared to 8 inches in men. Plus, the urethra opening in women lies close to the vagina and anus, both bacteria-laden areas. Unfortunately, women's risk increases after menopause, since the drop in estrogen leads to

Watch out for bladder irritants

When you have a UTI, avoid coffee, spicy foods, and alcohol, which can irritate your bladder. And drink plenty of fluids to flush bacteria out of your urinary tract.

changes in the urinary tract, bladder, and immune system that make it harder to fight off infections.

Although men may not be as prone to UTIs, the infections are usually more serious and require longer drug treatment than in women. That's because, in men, the infection can spread to the prostate gland, and bacterial prostate infections are much harder to treat and cure.

A frequent urge to urinate, pain and burning during urination, cloudy or reddish urine, and a general sense of feeling bad all over are classic signs of a UTI. Seniors, however, may have none of these symptoms. Instead, they may experience stomach pain, nausea, vomiting, confusion, coughing, or shortness of breath. You won't normally run a fever with a UTI, but you may if the infection has spread to your kidneys.

Doctors treat most UTIs with antibiotics to wipe out the offending bacteria. Other drugs can relieve pain and burning while the antibiotics do their job. Applying a heating pad may help, too. The best natural treatment is prevention. Establishing good bathroom habits and choosing your clothes wisely go a long way to warding off infections.

- Always wipe from front to back if you're a woman to avoid contaminating the urethra with bacteria from stool.
- Avoid wearing tight-fitting pants and skip nylon panties in favor of cotton-crotch underwear and stockings. Wash underwear with mild detergents.

- Stop using feminine hygiene sprays and scented douches, especially if you have sensitive skin. Both irritate the urethra. Plus, douching may kill antiviral organisms that naturally live in your vagina, making you more susceptible to the human papillomavirus (HPV) linked to cervical cancer.
- Wash your genital area with mild soapy water after bowel movements, and take showers instead of baths when possible.

Tart treat wipes out infections

Native Americans first taught the Pilgrims the value of cranberries for bladder and kidney problems, and up until World War II, doctors used them regularly to treat urinary tract infections (UTIs). Now the berry is back in style, and experts say drinking just one or two glasses of its juice daily can prevent painful UTIs.

Proanthocyanidins, the same compounds that make cranberries red, also keep bacteria from sticking to the walls of your urinary tract. If they can't hold on, they get washed out by the flow of urine and never have the chance to establish an infection. That's especially good news if you get frequent UTIs. Research suggests bacteria have an easier time clinging to bladder walls in women prone to recurrent bladder infections. Regular cranberry therapy could help turn this tide.

Experts typically recommend drinking 8 to 16 ounces of pure cranberry juice every day. You'll need even more if you drink cranberry juice cocktail. Eating about one-third cup of dried, sweetened

Lower your risk of UTIs

Just like good bathroom habits, practicing good sexual hygiene can lower your incidence of urinary tract infections. Always wash your genital area and urinate both before and after sex to empty your bladder and flush bacteria out of your urethra.

cranberries or taking a 300-to 400-milligram cranberry supplement twice daily may boast the same protective benefits as juice.

Cranberries may help prevent infections, but no solid evidence shows they can treat existing UTIs, so see your doctor if you think you have one. Also, talk to your doctor before trying cranberry therapy if you have a history of oxalate kidney stones or take the blood-thinning drug warfarin (Coumadin).

Friendly dairy fights bad bacteria

Eating yogurt, cheese, kefir, and other fermented dairy products may break the cycle of recurrent UTIs in women by building up the number of beneficial, or probiotic, bacteria living in the vagina. Premenopausal women who indulged in these treats at least three times a week were 80 percent less likely to get a urinary tract infection than women who ate them less than once a week in a recent Finnish study.

Before menopause, your vagina is naturally home to *lactobacilli*, a family of friendly bacteria, like *acidophilus*. They crowd out bad bacteria and produce lactic acid, which the bad bugs behind UTIs can't live in. After menopause, your natural levels of vaginal *lactobacilli* drop, thanks to a drop in estrogen. Experts think that's one reason women tend to get more UTIs after menopause.

Eating probiotic foods, like yogurt, or taking certain probiotic supplements may help restore that bacterial balance. Look for foods and supplements that claim to contain *L. rhamnosus GR-1* and *L. casei GR-1*, two specific strains of *Lactobacillus* that have shown promise protecting against UTIs in studies.

Talk to your doctor before starting probiotic therapy if you have cancer, diabetes, or take immune-suppressing drugs, and let your doctors know you use probiotics before undergoing surgery.

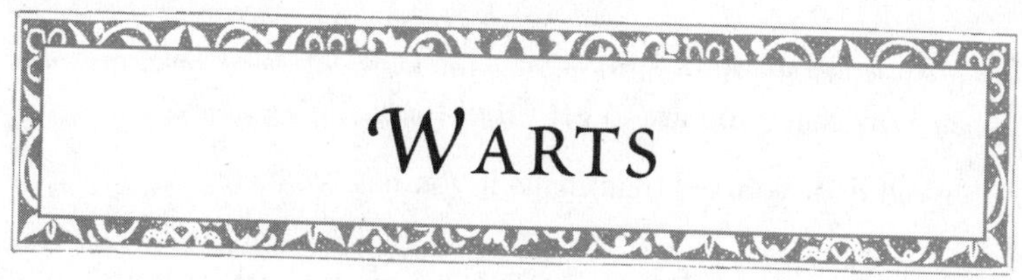

Warts

Trade old-time cures for new home treatments

When English politician Oliver Cromwell asked his portrait artist to paint him "warts and all," he expressed a common opinion about warts. They're ugly, and most people would rather not have them. But the reality, as Cromwell pointed out, is that people do get this common skin infection. A strain of the human papillomavirus (HPV) causes warts, and they can appear on your hands, feet, face, or other areas. Other types of HPV are linked to cervical cancer. Warts can be smooth or rough, large bumps or nearly flat, dark or pink. They're most common in children and teens, but people of all ages can get them.

No doubt you've heard of many old-time cures for warts, from dousing them with vinegar to tying on a banana peel or even rubbing them with a penny. Your warts may go away after you try these tricks, but it may be due to the power of suggestion. If you believe rubbing your warts with a potato slice will heal them, then your body may make it happen. Some doctors still use this "suggestive therapy" on children, who believe in the penny cure or the banana remedy. Since warts usually go away within months to two years without treatment, it's hard to argue that these folksy cures aren't real. Here are some things to remember:

- If your wart doesn't hurt, it's probably best to let it be. Even the toughest treatments don't always work, and some therapies can cause pain or scarring.

- Warts can spread, and they can be painful on the soles of your feet. These "plantar" warts look a lot like calluses. See a doctor if a plantar wart hurts when you walk.

- It's best to avoid home remedies for warts on your face, no matter how eager you are to get rid of them.
- Avoid do-it-yourself treatments if you have diabetes.

The HPV virus is all around, and you can pick it up by walking barefoot outdoors or near public showers or pools. Wear sandals or flip-flops to steer clear of the germs. If you're one of the unlucky people prone to getting warts, have your favorite home remedy ready. You'll probably get them again. If nothing else works, your doctor can treat your warts with liquid nitrogen, laser therapy, or by cutting them out.

Smart, easy ways to banish warts

Don't forget to check your local pharmacy – or even your kitchen – before spending time and money on a doctor's visit. You may get good results from these over-the-counter and natural remedies.

Do it yourself. Home treatments like Compound W or Dr. Scholl's Clear Away contain salicylic acid, which slowly dissolves the wart. Soak your wart in warm water for five minutes, then dry it off before you apply the treatment. You'll probably need to use it every day until your wart is gone, but experts say it works on 75 percent of warts – even better than liquid nitrogen.

Give garlic a go. Rubbing with a cut clove of raw garlic is an old-time trick for getting rid of warts, and it may work. Researchers tested applying either a watery or a fatty garlic extract on warts twice each day. Within two weeks, most warts treated with the fatty garlic extract had disappeared. The watery garlic extract didn't work as quickly, but it banished many warts within two months. Experts think garlic kills the virus that causes warts or possibly boosts your immune system to fight back. Raw garlic can cause a rash on some people, so protect the skin around your wart if you try this trick.

Pick a papaya. Papain, an enzyme in papaya, works like a "biological scalpel" to dissolve dead tissue. It's an old folk remedy for warts, boils, and ringworm. Try rubbing the juice of a green papaya, or papaw, on your wart several times a day.

Duct tape: simple solution or crazy cure?

Freezing therapy can hurt, and putting a liquid on your wart every day is a pain. A simple, cheap way to clear up children's warts would sure make parents happy. Maybe that's why duct tape occlusion therapy (DTOT) has grown so popular. Question is – does it work?

Researchers in Washington state tested duct tape on children, comparing DTOT with cryotherapy (freezing with liquid nitrogen). Duct tape worked better than freezing, usually within the first four weeks. But in a second study, on schoolchildren in the Netherlands, DTOT didn't work as well. The duct tape helped shrink some warts and banish others, but it didn't work much better than a placebo (fake treatment). Some experts think this second study was too small and not planned well, however.

Here's how duct tape therapy works.

- Cut a piece of duct tape the size of your wart, and place it over the wart. Leave the tape in place for seven days. If it falls off, replace it with a new piece.
- On the evening of the seventh day, remove the tape and soak your wart in warm water for five minutes. Afterward, rub it gently with a pumice stone.
- The next morning, apply a new piece of duct tape. Repeat the cycle until your wart disappears.

Even people who believe DTOT works don't understand what is going on, but they think the tape irritates your skin. That might kick start your immune system into battling the wart.

WEIGHT GAIN

Clever ways to cut calories

Everybody is doing it. In a recent Gallup poll, six in 10 Americans admitted they have tried to lose weight. The key word is "tried." If you're dieting, you know how tough losing those love handles can be. The benefits are worth it, though – a longer life with fewer health problems.

Simply trying to lose weight saves lives, says the Centers for Disease Control. People who try in vain to drop pounds are still more likely to live than people who never even give it a go. Those who succeed reap big rewards, too.

- Slimming down is the single most effective way to lower your triglycerides, plus it ups your "good" HDL cholesterol and slashes "bad" LDL cholesterol.
- Shedding as few as five to 10 pounds may even drop your high blood pressure enough for you to stop taking medication.
- Trimming just a few calories a day could thwart age-related damage throughout your body and add years to your life. Being overweight, however, starts slowing your memory in middle age and may raise your risk of dementia.

As with everything, there's a good and bad way to shape up. These hints can help you reach your goal of a slimmer, trimmer you.

Go slow and steady. The best way to slim down and stay that way is to aim for a slow, steady rate of weight loss. The gradual change may not feel as rewarding as suddenly dropping a lot of pounds, but you're much more likely to stay slim and trim, and much less likely to suffer with gallstones and other side effects of rapid weight loss.

Set realistic goals. Don't aim to lose more than 10 percent of your body weight, at least at first. You may be tempted to give up if the goal seems too hard to reach. Plus, cutting too many calories can actually slow your metabolism, making it tough to shed those pounds.

Try the buddy system. Enlist the aid of your spouse, partner, or best friend. Invite them to join your diet if they need to lose weight. Sticking to your guns – and your weight loss plan – is easier with moral support and a sympathetic ear. Plus, being on the same eating plan as your partner simplifies shopping and cooking, and you won't be tempted to poach naughty foods from their plate.

Keep a diary. Use it to log your daily food and activities. Many studies show tracking your food and exercise habits will help you lose weight and keep it off. Also, note your weekly weigh-ins. Seeing your progress in black and white will motivate you during the tough times, and you may discover patterns of eating and behavior that have kept you overweight all these years.

To lose weight, your body will have to use up more energy than it gets from food. Scientists measure food energy in calories. If you eat more calories than you use up during the day, you gain weight. If you burn off more calories than you eat, either by exercising more or simply eating less, you lose weight. It doesn't have to be hard. You can find effective, natural ways – right in your own home – to help you shed the pounds. Read on for simple tricks to cut down and burn off calories.

Feel full on less food

Some foods practically force your body to lose weight. Eight to try are whole-grain bread, soup, apples, oranges, broccoli, lentils, brown rice, and Canadian bacon. The secret – they help you feel full while adding fewer calories to your diet.

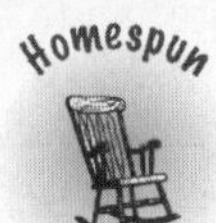

Pantry staple nixes sweet tooth

Turn off your craving for sweets and help melt off the pounds with this easy weight-loss secret. The next time your insatiable sweet tooth kicks in, just put this common household item on your tongue. Dissolve a teaspoon of baking soda in warm water, swish it around like mouthwash, then spit it out.

Fill up on fiber. Results are in from a study of 27,000 people – eat whole grains if you want to lose weight. Eating more whole-grain foods, especially those made with bran, kept men slimmer over the course of eight years. The more they ate, the less weight they gained. What's more, other research shows choosing whole grains over refined ones actually helps you lose weight.

Whole grains are rich in fiber, and experts think filling up on high-fiber foods helps you eat less throughout the day. They pack fewer calories per ounce than foods made with refined grains, like white flour or white rice, and they satisfy hunger better, to boot. This double-diet whammy is the perfect way to lose weight without going hungry.

Choose foods made with bran, and check food labels for whole grain ingredients, including "whole oats" and "cracked wheat." Consider drinking a glass of orange juice with a psyllium fiber supplement, like Fiberall, stirred in 30 minutes before every meal, and you'll be well on the way to a slimmer you.

Save room for soup. It's the one food you can eat and eat and still lose weight. Soup is a low energy-dense food, meaning a single cup contains fewer calories than most other foods. It also takes up a lot of room in your stomach, so it satisfies hunger better. Eating two servings every day of soup helped dieters lose 50 percent more weight than eating other snacks with the same number of calories.

The soup-slurpers felt fuller throughout the day, which may have helped them snack less.

Skip the cream-based soups, which are heavy on fat and high in calories. Instead, enjoy those with a vegetable- or chicken-broth base and loaded with high-fiber foods like brown rice, vegetables, and lentils. And try to eat more fruits and vegetables with high water, fiber, and nutrient content, such as apples or broccoli.

Pile on the protein. Eating a little lean protein with breakfast could keep you full until lunch. In a Purdue University study, adding a slice of Canadian bacon to their breakfast helped overweight women feel less hungry for four hours than those who skipped the protein. This nutrient makes your body release the hunger-reducing hormone PYY, so you snack less during the day.

Eat slowly. It does help you eat less. Experts gave two groups of college women the same meal but told one group to eat fast and the other to chew each bite 15 to 20 times. The slow-eaters not only ate 67 fewer calories, but they also felt fuller than the fast-eaters for an hour afterward.

5 smart ways to win the snack battle

Low fat! Made with real fruit! Food labels on every kind of snack scream about their goodness. Unfortunately, some so-called healthy food can lead to weight gain as easily as the junk it replaces in your pantry.

Take low-fat foods. You may think since they're lower in fat, they are also much lower in calories. In reality, they typically contain only 30 fewer calories per serving than their regular-fat counterparts. However, people in one study ate nearly 30 percent more when they knew they were eating a low-fat snack. Overweight people ate almost 50 percent more. Mistakes like these can ruin your diet. These five rules can help save it.

- Read the nutrition labels on food. Look for snacks with the most nutrients and the fewest calories, and check both the sugar and fat content.
- Grab several brands of the same item when shopping, and choose the one with the fewest calories, not just the least fat.
- Check the serving size on the nutrition label. Sometimes manufacturers try to make a food's nutrition numbers look better (less fat or fewer calories) by basing them on ridiculously small servings.
- Make sure good-for-you foods like vegetables weren't prepared with butter, cream, or breading.
- Choose naturally low-fat, nutrient-rich foods like fresh, unprocessed fruits and vegetables over processed, prepackaged "healthy" snacks.

Easy tricks to eating less

Drop pounds without dieting or even consciously watching what you eat. You can actually trick yourself into eating less by making small portions of food look bigger.

Years of study show it's not how much you eat that makes you feel full but how much you think you have eaten. By fooling your eyes into seeing portions as larger than they actually are, you can fool your stomach into feeling full with less food. Experts say trimming just 15 to 20 percent of your daily calories this way could help you lose 30 pounds in a year, with little effort.

Downsize your dishes. Use smaller plates and bowls at home. Bigger dishes create an optical illusion, so a normal-sized scoop of food that fills a small plate looks lost on a big one. If a portion looks too small to your eyes, your stomach assumes it is, prompting you to eat more.

Even food experts fall for it. In one sneaky study, nutrition experts ate 30 percent more ice cream when they scooped it into extra-large

Good giggle fights flab

The next time you're deciding what to watch on TV, opt for a comedy. You burn 20 percent more calories while laughing than when not. Having a good hoot for 15 minutes burns up to 40 calories, enough for a piece of chocolate. Laugh like that every day for a year, and you could lose 4.4 pounds – no joke.

bowls than they did using regular-sized bowls. Similarly, when you serve yourself from a huge bowl or platter, you tend to take and eat more food than usual. Try substituting salad plates for your regular plates and serving meals from smaller platters and bowls.

Shrink your spoons. The size of your utensils matters, too. The ice cream-eating researchers dished up almost 15 percent more when they used large scoops compared to small ones. In another study, people were allowed to serve themselves as many M&M candies as they wanted. Halfway through the study, researchers swapped the small serving spoon in the bowl with a large one. People who used the big spoon ate twice as much candy. So while trading in your big dishes, hunt for smaller silverware, too, and make a point of serving meals with smaller spoons, scoops, and forks.

Go skinny with glasses. Drink high-calorie beverages like soda and alcohol from tall, slim glasses rather than short, wide ones, and you will automatically drink about 30 percent less. Short, wide glasses look like they hold less, so you tend to pour more into them than you think.

Plump up your food. The way you prepare the food you eat can trick your stomach just as surely as the size plates you use. People who normally ate a half-pound hamburger were given a quarter-pound burger dressed up with lots of lettuce, onion, and tomatoes to make it look as big as the half-pound burger. These hungry people

Calcium crucial to weight loss

Rapid weight loss seems to speed up osteoporosis in post-menopausal women. Talk to your doctor about taking calcium and vitamin D supplements to prevent bone loss if you are on an extreme weight-loss diet.

felt just as full after eating the smaller burger as they did after eating the big one, but they consumed many fewer calories. Whipping foods to make them fuller and thicker has the same stomach-fooling effect.

Secret to burning fat faster

Dieting is well and good, but to lose weight and keep it off, you must exercise, too. That's your secret weapon. The more muscle you have, the more calories you'll burn even when you're just watching TV. Plus, exercise helps prevent osteoporosis, especially if you are dieting. Cutting back on calories without adding in exercise leads to bone loss in your hip and spine. Try this advice to supercharge your workouts and help those pounds melt away.

Do something you enjoy. Working out doesn't have to mean gym memberships and aerobic classes. It can mean yard work, yoga, and a daily walk. Find an exercise you enjoy or that makes you feel accomplished, then stick with it until it becomes habit. Your body and mind will get "addicted" in a good way, and you won't want to miss a day.

Invest in weights. Strength training halts the middle-age spread of your waistline. It builds muscle, which in turn, helps you burn more calories. In fact, a study showed that overweight, middle-aged women who lifted weights just twice a week became stronger and did not gain weight as they aged, the opposite of what happens to most people. In particular, these women lost belly fat, which lowered their risk of heart disease.

Your muscles need new challenges to keep growing, much like your brain. Alternate which muscles you work each day – legs one day, arms and back the next – and avoid working the same ones two days in a row. Gradually add more repetitions and increase the amount of weight you lift.

Get your heart pumping. The heart is a muscle, too. Keep it in tip-top shape with aerobic activities that get your heart rate up, like brisk walking, dancing, and swimming. Swap out activities regularly. If you swim one day, then walk or jog the next. Boost the benefit even more by slowing down for five minutes, then speeding up for five minutes.

Women should aim for a moderate, but not intense, aerobic workout. Strenuous activity actually whets women's appetites, prompting them to eat more. Moderate activity doesn't. In one study, women who did moderate aerobic workouts lost more weight than those who trained intensely. Men don't have this problem. The harder they exercise, the more calories they burn.

Keep moving. Exercise will only do so much. If you walk for 30 minutes but spend the rest of the day watching TV, you won't lose weight. It's OK to relax, but stay active throughout the day as much as possible to maximize your weight loss. You'll drop those pounds in no time.

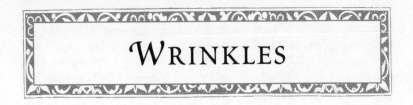

Wrinkles

Smooth solutions for the lines of time

"Wrinkles should merely indicate where smiles have been," wrote Mark Twain at age 62. Not everyone accepts aging with such grace. Folk medicine is full of tricks to prevent and cure crow's feet and eyebrow furrows – like holding a raw potato to your skin, or avoiding prunes. Science doesn't put much stock in these ideas, but scientists will say wrinkles are caused by a combination of time, gravity, and too much fun in the sun. Smoking can make them worse, while losing weight quickly can make them more noticeable.

Here's how it works. As you age, the network of collagen and elastin fibers that gives skin its structure starts to unravel. Skin stretches and sags instead of bouncing back. Meanwhile, you lose fat where you might like to keep it – in your face and hands. Your skin makes less oil and cells renew themselves more slowly. All that adds up to a big change in your skin over the years.

To slow time's march across your face, doctors can offer face lifts, injections of filler materials, laser therapy, and many other pricey and painful treatments. But there's a lot you can do without spending tons of money or time recovering from the scalpel.

- Stay out of the sun. Photoaging, or damage from the sun, is the biggest cause of wrinkled skin. It's never too late to start protecting yourself. Use sunscreen, wear a hat and protective clothing, and stay indoors when the sun is brightest. See the *Sunburn* chapter for more on defending your skin and dealing with age spots.

- Don't smoke. It makes your skin age faster by producing cell-damaging free radicals and enzymes linked to wrinkles.

- Stay hydrated. Drink plenty of water to keep your skin plump and full of moisture.
- Wash wisely. Don't use tap water on your face more than once a day since it strips oil and moisture from your skin. And instead of harsh soaps, use a mild one containing a moisturizer. See the *Dry skin* chapter to learn about ways to help this skin problem.
- Exercise daily. It will keep blood flowing to your skin.
- Sleep on your back. Keep gravity from working overtime.
- Lower your stress level. That means don't worry so much – even about wrinkles.

Feel-good diet can turn back the clock

The fountain of youth overflows with a stream of olive oil and other staples – all part of something called the Mediterranean diet. This simple eating regimen includes plenty of fish, whole grains, fruits, vegetables, and, of course, olive oil, but little red meat, butter, and sweets. Experts believe following this kind of diet leads to less skin aging and wrinkles.

Researchers, Dr. Mark Wahlqvist and Dr. Antigone Kouris-Blazos, studied more than 450 seniors, both fair- and dark-skinned, living from Sweden to Australia to Greece. They compared diets and skin condition, noting sun damage and wrinkles. Surprisingly, people with eating habits that included the traditionally healthy foods of the

No more funny faces

The American Academy of Dermatology says don't bother with facial exercises that claim to strengthen the muscles in your face and make you look younger. Repeated facial movements – among other things – actually cause wrinkles and fine lines.

Mediterranean diet had younger-looking skin – regardless of climate or heritage.

So what is going on? Antioxidant foods – like vegetables with lots of vitamins C, A, and E – and certain fats – like those in fish and olive oil – protect skin cells and prevent early wrinkling and aging. They help your skin heal from free radicals that attack your collagen and elastin tissue. It's interesting that people in the study with the least skin damage also avoided saturated fats and sugars.

Of course, a lifetime of this diet is best, but it's never too late to improve your food choices. Try for at least five servings of vegetables each day, including choices like leafy greens, asparagus, spinach, and eggplant, along with fruits like prunes, cherries, and apples. Eat a serving of fish a bit bigger than a deck of cards twice a week, and cut back on red meats, butter, whole-fat dairy foods, and sweets. Both your skin and your heart will thank you.

Best bets for younger-looking skin

Your grandmother might have tried to rub out her wrinkles with goose grease, but you can do better. Check any drugstore and you'll find dozens of lotions and creams that promise to banish all signs of aging. What ingredients really work?

Add some AHA. Alpha hydroxy acids (AHAs) help peel off the top layer of dead skin cells to make way for fresh new cells.

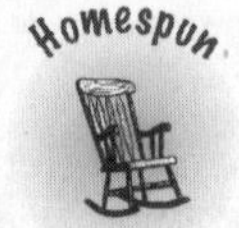

Surprising way to wake up your face

Hemorrhoid cream is an old-time remedy for wrinkles, puffy eyes, and a saggy jaw. It constricts blood vessels and shrinks tissues – wherever you put it. Try a dab under your puffy eyes or on those stubborn forehead lines. Nobody else needs to know what's on the label of your secret aging antidote.

AHAs such as glycolic acid can be up to 10 percent strength in over-the-counter creams and higher strengths with a prescription.

Count on coenzyme Q10. Also known as ubiquinone or CoQ10, this is an antioxidant made naturally in your body – but less and less as you age and with exposure to sunlight. It helps reduce your risk of sun damage and wrinkles, so it's a common ingredient in anti-aging creams.

Don't forget your C. Like other antioxidants, vitamin C fights sun damage to skin cells. In a cream, it helps your skin rebuild collagen. Early versions were unstable, so the vitamin C would break down quickly and turn the cream yellow. Newer formulas keep their strength over time.

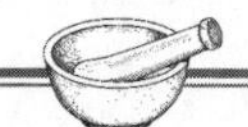

Who says having egg on your face is reason to blush? Try this low-cost, facial mask to make fine lines less noticeable. Mix together 1 tablespoon honey, 1 egg white, 1 teaspoon glycerin – from your local drug or beauty stores – plus about 1/4 cup flour. Spread this paste onto your face and throat. Relax for 10 minutes, then rinse off gently.

Keep retinoids in mind. These topical forms of vitamin A include the prescription drug tretinoin (Retin-A), first used for acne and now found quite helpful for smoothing wrinkles and boosting collagen production. Other vitamin A products include retinol, which you'll find in some over-the-counter skin creams. The more powerful retinoids can irritate your skin and make it more sensitive to the sun, so be sure to use sunscreen every day.

Don't expect dramatic changes, no matter what the active ingredient. A recent study comparing several common brands of anti-aging creams found even the best reduced wrinkle depth by less than 10 percent – hardly noticeable. If you want to save a few bucks on certain skincare products, some experts say try a men's version. Often they contain the same active ingredients at a lower price.

YEAST INFECTIONS

Tips to soothe the savage yeast

You may know the signs – itching and redness in your vaginal area, burning when you urinate, and a white, cheesy discharge. You've got it – a yeast infection. About three-quarters of all women get at least one yeast infection, and some are struck repeatedly with this itchy curse. It's an inconvenience, and it can get in the way of your active lifestyle.

Candida albicans, the type of fungus that causes most vaginal yeast infections, normally lives in your healthy body. It loves warm, dark, moist places, and it usually causes no problems. But *Candida* can grow out of control to cause a troublesome infection at certain times, like when your body is weakened from stress or a bad diet. Taking antibiotics to fight infections can upset your body's normal bacterial balance, giving yeast the chance to multiply. A high level of the female hormone estrogen – from birth-control pills, pregnancy, or hormone-replacement therapy – can also give *Candida* a foothold. Some people think a diet with lots of sugar is another cause of yeast infections. In fact, repeated yeast infections can be a sign of diabetes.

To help a yeast infection heal and keep it from coming back, follow these good-hygiene guidelines from the American College of Obstetricians and Gynecologists.

- Keep your genital area clean and dry.
- Avoid tight-fitting pants or pantyhose without a cotton crotch.
- Wear cotton – not nylon – underwear.
- Stay away from perfumed soap and scented toilet paper.

- Don't use pads or tampons with deodorant or plastic coatings.
- Skip feminine sprays and talc products.
- Avoid tight-fitting clothing while you sleep.

Your doctor may prescribe antifungal drugs to treat a serious yeast infection or preventive drugs to avoid future infections. If you have experienced yeast infections before and know the signs, you can try an over-the-counter antifungal drug like Monistat or Gyne-Lotrimin. Some brands are available in seven-day, three-day, and even one-day versions. The longer courses of treatment seem to work better. Whether or not you use drugs to prevent or treat yeast infections, try the following do-it-yourself solutions to keep the yeast beast at bay.

Yogurt KOs yeast in biological battle

Veteran sufferers of yeast infections seek out ways to avoid a future bout with this itchy curse. One trick that's been around for a century is eating yogurt to fight the yeast.

The idea of using probiotics, or certain strains of friendly bacteria, to fight disease is nothing new. Some experts say not having the right balance of "good" germs can lead to many health problems, including irritable bowel syndrome, respiratory infections, and bad breath.

In the case of yeast infection, certain bacteria strains found in yogurt, including *Lactobacillus acidophilus,* may control the overgrowth of *Candida* fungi. These bugs produce lactic acid, which creates an unfriendly place for yeast to live. One study found that women eating 8 ounces of yogurt with *Lactobacillus* every day had fewer yeast infections during the six-month test period. In fact, some women who had good results from eating yogurt refused to switch to the non-yogurt group when it was their turn. Other trials showed weaker results for yogurt eaters, but experts aren't giving up on yogurt just yet. This kind of probiotic therapy is harmless and may help you avoid a future yeast infection.

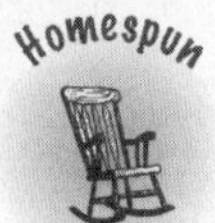

Sit a spell in a salty vinegar bath

Yeast infections are nothing new, so women have thought up some inventive ways of dealing with the problem. A vinegar-and-salt sitz bath is an old standby. Salt relieves the itching, while vinegar may keep the yeast in check. Try this half-half-half recipe. Fill your bathtub halfway with warm water, then pour in a half cup of salt and a half cup of vinegar. Enjoy your soothing soak for about a half hour. But don't use vinegar solution in a douche. Experts say douching is unnecessary and can lead to infections.

Look for yogurt that proclaims "live active yogurt cultures" on the label. Brands like Stonyfield Farm and Dannon Activia yogurt or DanActive yogurt drink are good choices. Along with your friendly bugs, you'll also get calcium and other nutrients.

4 get-tough ways to kill Candida

Candida fungus from a yeast infection can live on your underwear, and regular laundering may not be powerful enough to kill it. You need to get your undies clean to avoid reinfection. Try these get-tough ideas to kill *Candida* that may be hiding on your unmentionables.

- Scrub the crotch of your panties with unscented detergent before you put them in the washing machine.
- Boil your undies to kill off the fungus. Then wash them with unscented detergent.
- Soak your underwear in a bleach solution before you put them in the washer, or use bleach during laundering.
- Touch a hot iron to cotton underwear to kill yeast.

HEALING HERBS

Herb	Condition or symptom	Effectiveness rating
alfalfa	diabetes	★★
	heart disease	★★
	inflammation	★
aloe vera juice	constipation	★★★
berberine	diabetes	★★
	high cholesterol	★★
bromelain	inflammation	★★★
	rheumatoid arthritis	★★
chamomile	insomnia	★★
	skin inflammation	★★
dandelion	diabetes	★★
	inflammation	★★
devil's claw	back pain	★★★
	inflammation	★
	osteoarthritis	★★★
elder	inflammation	★
eyebright	inflammation	★★
fennel	constipation	★
	gas, abdominal cramps	★
feverfew	inflammation	★
	migraine headaches	★★★
	rheumatoid arthritis	★★
flaxseed	constipation	★★★
	high blood pressure	★★
garlic	athlete's foot	★
	high blood pressure	★★
ginger	headache	★
	motion sickness	★★
	nausea	★★

HEALING HERBS (CONTINUED)

Herb	Condition or symptom	Effectiveness rating
ginseng	diabetes	★★★
	inflammation	★
goldenseal	inflammation	★
green tea	diabetes	★★
	heart disease	★★
	high blood pressure	★★
lavender	anxiety	★★★
	inflammation	★
peppermint	tension headache	★★
	irritable bowel syndrome	★★★
psyllium	constipation	★★★
	high cholesterol	★★★
	irritable bowel syndrome	★★
St. John's wort	depression (mild to moderate)	★★★
	inflammation	★
turmeric	diabetes	★
	inflammation	★★
	osteoarthritis	★★

Effectiveness ratings are based on how much research has been done on the herbs as treatments for each condition or symptom.

★★★ – Remedy has strong scientific evidence it works.
★★ – Remedy has weak scientific evidence it works.
★ – Traditional remedy has little scientific evidence.

Before you use an herbal supplement, be sure it's safe. Some herbs are dangerous for people with certain health conditions, and others don't mix well with drugs. For detailed information about a particular herb, see the list of herb and drug interactions at the U.S. government's Web site, *www.medlineplus.gov*. Select "Drugs & Supplements," then find your desired herb in the alphabetical list.

Index

A

B

C

D

E

F

G

H

I

K

L

M

N

O

P

Q

R

S

T

U

V

W

X

Y

Z